CHILDHOOD OBESITY

Ethical and Policy Issues

Kristin Voigt, Stuart G. Nicholls,
and Garrath Williams

OXFORD
UNIVERSITY PRESS

OXFORD
UNIVERSITY PRESS

Oxford University Press is a department of the University of
Oxford. It furthers the University's objective of excellence in research,
scholarship, and education by publishing worldwide.

Oxford   New York
Auckland   Cape Town   Dar es Salaam   Hong Kong   Karachi
Kuala Lumpur   Madrid   Melbourne   Mexico City   Nairobi
New Delhi   Shanghai   Taipei   Toronto

With offices in
Argentina   Austria   Brazil   Chile   Czech Republic   France   Greece
Guatemala   Hungary   Italy   Japan   Poland   Portugal   Singapore
South Korea   Switzerland   Thailand   Turkey   Ukraine   Vietnam

Oxford is a registered trademark of Oxford University Press
in the UK and certain other countries.

Published in the United States of America by
Oxford University Press
198 Madison Avenue, New York, NY 10016

Library of Congress Cataloging-in-Publication Data
Voigt, Kristin, 1979– author.
Childhood obesity : ethical and policy issues / Kristin Voigt, Stuart G. Nicholls, and Garrath Williams.
p. ; cm.
Includes bibliographical references.
ISBN 978–0–19–996448–2 (hardcover : alk. paper)
I. Nicholls, Stuart G., author.   II. Williams, Garrath, author.   III. Title.
[DNLM: 1. Obesity.   2. Child.   3. Ethics.   4. Health Education.   5. Health Policy.
WD 210]
RJ399.C6
618.92'398—dc23   2013028115

9 8 7 6 5 4 3 2 1
Printed in the United States of America
on acid-free paper

CONTENTS

ACKNOWLEDGMENTS

We are grateful to many people for their support and feedback while writing this book.

For comments and feedback on different chapters, we would like to thank Karin Bammann, Sam Clark, Unna Danner, Francis Fallon, John Foster, Mairi Levitt, Wencke Gwozdz, Lucia Reisch, and Dita Wickins-Drazilova, as well as colleagues at a philosophy work-in-progress session at Lancaster University. We are also grateful to two anonymous referees for Oxford University Press for comments on draft chapters. For further discussions, advice, and input, we would like to thank David Archard, Ilse De Bourdeaudhuij, Ruth Chadwick, Lauren Lissner, Ginny Newsham, Kerry O'Brien, Justin Sherwin, Rhonda Smith, Delfien Van Dyck, and Myfanwy Williams. We would also like to thank Isaac Stethem for his assistance with collation of the manuscript and for curating articles in (often confusing) reference management software.

A large part of the work on this book was undertaken as part of the IDEFICS study (Identification and prevention of Dietary- and lifestyle-induced health EFfects In Children and infantS). We gratefully acknowledge the financial support of the European Community within the Sixth RTD Framework Program Contract No. 016181 (FOOD). Garrath Williams has also undertaken some of the work presented here as part of the I.Family Study (http://www.ifamilystudy.eu). He gratefully acknowledges the financial support of the European Community within the Seventh RTD Framework Program Contract No. 266044.

We are also extremely grateful to members of the IDEFICS and I.Family studies for sharing their expertise, findings, and enthusiasm with us. For their support and encouragement throughout, we would like to record our thanks to the coordinator of IDEFICS and I.Family, Wolfgang Ahrens, as well as to Iris Pigeot as deputy coordinator of both studies, and to Alfonso Siani as deputy coordinator of I.Family. Special thanks go also to Ina Alvarez. We should emphasize that the views expressed here are strictly those of the authors, and not of other scientists who have collaborated on these research projects.

Kristin Voigt would like to thank her friends and colleagues at McGill for providing a wonderful work environment during the completion of the manuscript. She is very grateful to her family for their support and encouragement throughout this project. Kristin also gratefully acknowledges financial support from the Canadian Institutes for Health Research.

Stuart Nicholls would like to thank Brenda Wilson, Jamie Brehaut, and Rebecca Nicholls for their flexibility, support, and enduring assistance and for allowing time to complete the manuscript. And thank you to all who provided input and comments on posters, presentations, and manuscripts that have informed the content of this book.

Garrath Williams wishes to thank Ruth Chadwick, Robert Geyer, Morris Kaplan, Veronika Koller, Mairi Levitt, Andrew Quick, and Linda Woodhead for their support and encouragement. He is very grateful to the Department of Intercultural Communication and Management at Copenhagen Business School for providing a collegial and supportive environment during the completion of the manuscript—special thanks to Wencke Gwozdz, Lucia Reisch, Dorte Salskov-Iversen, and Majbritt Vendelbo.

INTRODUCTION

Obesity as an Object of Concern

Increasing rates of overweight and obesity have become a major concern in many high-income countries across the world. There has been a notable rise in rates among adults, sparking research and interventions by health professionals and corresponding media and political debate. However, concern about childhood obesity has been even more marked. In the US, estimates suggest that around 17 percent of children and adolescents may be obese (Ogden et al., 2012). Within Europe the prevalence of obesity has seen a huge increase over the last decades, with studies indicating a trend of increasing weight among school-aged children (Lien et al., 2010). Comparisons of school-aged children suggest that up to 30 percent of children in some European countries are overweight and around 5 percent may be obese (Ahrens et al., 2011b; Lobstein & Frelut, 2003; Yngve et al., 2007). Although this book will focus on the developed world, it is also clear that childhood obesity is becoming more prevalent in the developing world, too (Finucane et al., 2011; Hossain et al., 2007; Wang & Lobstein, 2006).

One of our reasons for writing this book stems from a belief that there are both good and bad reasons for our social concern about obesity, especially in children, and that it is important to be clear about these reasons in order to respond appropriately.

On the one hand, there are well-justified fears that overweight and obesity bode ill for the future health of affected children. This may be because overweight and obesity directly damage the developing body, and some evidence speaks to this side of the story. Adiposity—high levels of body fat—seems to increase children's risks of health conditions such as type 2 diabetes, nonalcoholic fatty liver disease, orthopedic problems, and obstructive sleep apnea (Lobstein et al., 2010). In addition to the physiological effects, there are also concerns that obesity affects children's psychological well-being, for example in relation to self-esteem, feelings of loneliness, and depressive symptoms, particularly in girls (Erickson et al., 2000; Strauss, 2000). In addition, many of the commonly identified risk factors for overweight and obesity—such as low levels of physical fitness or unhealthy eating patterns—pose their own health risks, even for children who are not overweight. Increased rates of overweight and obesity should direct our attention toward unhealthy patterns of behavior found in many children's lives, regardless of their body weight or adiposity.

On the other hand, it is clear that modern Western societies are preoccupied with physical appearance, sexual attractiveness, and body image. As part of this, the fat body is highly stigmatized. To give just two initial illustrations: Leading campaigners on obesity still entertain large audiences with quips at the expense of the persons whom they claim to be concerned about. Thus one speaker at the 2011 European Congress on Obesity, "This is a condition where the problem enters the room before the patient does"—a line received with laughter rather than jeers. Psychologists have found that children of ever younger ages—as young as three, even—dislike associating with fatter children (Harriger et al., 2010), while many of their teachers and even health professionals share such stigmatizing attitudes (Neumark-Sztainer et al., 1999; O'Brien et al., 2006). In such a context, social and media concern about overweight and obesity should not be taken at face value, even when it is explicitly framed in health terms.

This is one reason why we will not speak in terms of a "battle against obesity." This is not just a squeamish distaste for military metaphors. When we consider the reasons that obesity prompts concern, obesity no longer looks like such a clear or simple target for our energies—let alone a military campaign. There are a complex set of health effects that may also appear in the absence of overweight or obesity and a complicated set of unhealthy behavior patterns that sometimes, but not always, result in overweight or obesity. Those behavior patterns have, in turn, many social, economic, and individual causes. As the so-called wars on "terror" or "drugs" should have taught us, wars against diffuse and hydra-headed targets cannot be won on their own terms. An underlying concern with the ill-health that is caused by, or associated with, obesity does not permit us to think in terms of a single clear problem.

More than this, widespread social concerns with body size and shape suggest that overweight and obesity are already far too much the objects of our enmity. Ask yourself the question: what more could Western societies do to persuade their members that the fatter body warrants dislike and should be brought back down to size? Nearly every popular magazine, every billboard, every film or television show tells us that the slim or muscular body is desirable—and the fat body is not. The fact is: we are already in the midst of a long "war against obesity." Clearly, this has not resulted in lower levels of overweight or obesity. But it has involved enormous misery for those affected.

This goes much beyond the ill-health that body fat may be associated with, to include the personal and social costs of stigma and discrimination. And it goes much beyond people who are or have been fat, to everyone whose relation to food is distorted by dieting or whose confidence in their bodies is damaged by fear or dislike of fat. As the number of overweight children increases and our cultural obsession with dieting and slimness grows, this misery will likely affect more and more children. Appeals for a (renewed) war against obesity have some of the notorious problems of attempts to "hate the sin but love the sinner." When darker forces of prejudice or disgust are in play, genuine concern for people's well-being can feed into stigmatizing and even punitive responses.

The "Child" in "Childhood Obesity"

If obesity is not a simple target for concern, the same is also true of childhood. There are good reasons to give especial attention to children and their healthy development. But there are also reasons to be cautious in our motivations and in the ways we respond to them.

Quite rightly, our children's situation attracts enormous concern: a society that fails to bring up children to become healthy, engaged, and responsible adults is simply a failing society. Clearly our societies are not failing in this way; but neither are they doing as well as we might hope. From the particular perspective of health and obesity, there are also special reasons to focus on children. We all know that prevention is better than cure. This is especially true in the case of obesity, where there are no clear cures and every putative remedy carries substantial costs and risks. There are also obvious reasons to regard preventing obesity in children as our best starting point. Because children are still growing, relative reductions in weight for height[1] can be achieved through weight maintenance and without drastic behavior changes (Doak et al., 2006). As habits are only beginning to take shape in childhood, it may be possible to prevent the formation of poor dietary habits and to inculcate patterns of healthy eating and physical activity. More broadly, the psychological capacities needed to take care of one's health are laid down in childhood.

But we should also keep in mind two reasons for caution when our concern focuses on children's situation. Sometimes concern for children can supplant

---

1. Usually gauged by reductions in body mass index or BMI—that is, body mass divided by the square of a person's height. We discuss some complexities in measurement in chapter 1.

proper consideration of what we owe our fellow adults. In most liberal societies, children's poverty or disadvantage is a more acceptable object of political concern than adults'.[2] We often rationalize this by regarding children as innocent while adults are seen as responsible for their situation. As we discuss in chapter 3, such claims are more complicated and difficult than they first appear, but one simple point can be made straightaway. If childhood really shapes future prospects and opportunities—which is the premise of so many interventions directed at children—then it cannot be right to assume that adults have effectively chosen their own fate and do not deserve assistance if they experience poverty or disadvantage. In our view, the same societies that fail many children also treat many adults unjustly. At the least, any social or political measure proposed to improve children's situation needs to be evaluated in terms of its effects on adults too—for example, on parents of lower socioeconomic status or single parents. And ideally, we believe, we should be formulating social policies to tackle poverty and disadvantage among adults as well. We will discuss socioeconomic injustice and weight stigma later in this book. Although our focus will remain on childhood, it needs to be kept in mind that these are issues affecting many adults as well.

In addition, concern for children's welfare often expresses itself in protective actions and policies. But protection is an ambiguous matter and often has a difficult relation to individual freedom and responsibility. Consider a playpen for an infant who has just learned to crawl or walk. From one perspective it is protective: it keeps the child within an area of safety. From another, it looks disturbingly like a cage: it restrains the child and limits his or her freedom. From yet another, it creates an area of freedom and empowerment: here the child has the power to move as he or she wishes, free from the hovering of an anxious parent who cannot yet trust the child with the risks posed by normal household objects. Arguably, none of these perspectives represents the whole truth. But the fact that the same practice can be looked at so differently should indicate that safety and freedom, empowerment and trust do not stand in simple relations. Protective measures may limit opportunities to learn, or fail to show trust in children who have already developed capacities of responsibility. In this situation, concerns for health and welfare can backfire. This is partly because they can restrict children's opportunities to become more independent or seem patronizing and overbearing to children themselves. It

---

2. It is no coincidence that the two recent First Ladies of Democrat presidents have turned their eye to children's situation. See Hillary Clinton (1996) and Michelle Obama's "Let's Move!" campaign, briefly discussed below.

is also because well-meaning restrictions can pose their own costs in terms of health. Thus one factor that has been associated with the increase in obesity and reduced levels of physical fitness in children is an increasing reluctance to grant children freedom from adult supervision, for example in getting to school or playing outdoors.[3]

We raise this issue at the start of this book in order to remind readers how little freedom children are already granted in modern societies. Initiatives to enhance safety, security, and surveillance as well as broader social changes, such as increased levels of traffic and reduced access to green spaces, often have the effect of restricting children's ability to be active, to relate to peers, and to use their own initiative. Whatever their other benefits, these restrictions and lost opportunities are likely to have costs in terms of obesity rates, physical fitness, and the development of independence and personal responsibility.

Some Limits to the Scope of This Book, and Why Our Discussion Ranges Broadly

This book concerns childhood obesity; moreover, it focuses principally on issues that belong to childhood as opposed to adolescence, before children really start to engage with adult rights and responsibilities. In addition to focusing on children's situation, this book also limits its attention to developed societies, above all, those of Europe, North America, and Australasia. These are not the only societies with increasing rates of childhood obesity. Societies that are developing industrial food infrastructures and creating food plenty for many of their members are also seeing take-offs in obesity rates. Nonetheless, developing countries face quite distinct issues, both in terms of the demography of obesity and in the political and institutional frameworks that may enable them to respond. While there are clearly lessons that they might learn from the Western experience—above all, that the abundance delivered by industrial agriculture and commercial food systems carries its own health risks and environmental costs—there is no simple way

---

3. This also seems to be a factor in another widespread developmental problem that has yet to attract public concern—the enormous increase in rates of short-sightedness in modern societies. See McCurdy et al. (2010, p. 110f) for a brief summary and further references, and Sherwin et al. (2012) for a review of evidence concerning the protective effect of outdoor activity against myopia.

to apply these lessons in such diverse demographic, economic, and political circumstances.[4]

For the most part, our aim is to explore and understand the many ethical and practical concerns raised by childhood obesity as a necessary precondition for reaching sensible agreements about how to proceed. This is another limit on our scope. Sometimes people assume that discussions of ethics and policy should issue in prescriptions for action. Of course, during our research on this topic, we have reached some judgments about appropriate responses by different actors, which we summarize in the book's conclusion.[5] However, even a reader who fully accepts our arguments and analyses may well disagree with our prescriptions for action, and we will mention shortly two important reasons why this should be. Accordingly, we do not see our task as that of providing a blueprint or shopping list of solutions. Instead, our main goal is to understand the complexity of the issues and the range of constructive responses that are available.

Even with these limitations in scope—children rather than adults or adolescents, developed rather than developing countries, exploring issues and options rather than propounding solutions—the book's task is not a simple one. The basic reason for this is that obesity is not a straightforward phenomenon. As we have mentioned and will continue to stress, obesity is symptomatic of broader health problems—such as metabolic syndrome and poor physical fitness—that also appear in many slim individuals, and do not appear in many fatter people. Like obesity, those problems arise from many causal factors. The contribution of each remains controversial and there is often no clean way to separate them from one another. We will discuss some of these complexities and the resulting controversies in chapter 1.

But obesity also raises much wider questions about how we organize our lives in contemporary societies, and how we think about our bodies, health, welfare, and freedom. This is because patterns of weight gain and ill-health are only partly caused by individual behaviors. For example, one contributory factor in the rise of obesity may be pollutants that affect some people's physiology in ways that lead them to gain body fat—so-called obesogens (Guthman,

---

4. For extended discussion of the social and political issues around chronic, noncommunicable diseases in developing as well as developed countries, see Stuckler and Siegel (2011). O'Dea and Eriksen (2010) also cover developing as well as developed countries.

5. For example, we believe that one of the most urgent tasks is to end stigma and discrimination against fatter people. One reason we feel able to endorse this prescription is because it represents a rare case of a practical judgment that can be acted on without cost to any other goal that is morally or politically important.

2011, ch. 5; Hatch et al., 2010; Trasande et al., 2012). More important still, how we each behave depends on an economic and social context that lends us some opportunities and closes off others—partly in terms of social norms or ideals, and partly by the incentives and costs attached to different choices. This is the "obesogenic environment" that we discuss in chapter 6.

Although the causal contributions remain controversial, most researchers agree that significant levels of obesity are to be expected in societies that tightly limit opportunities for physical activity and sustain food plenty through an industrial[6] and commercial food infrastructure.[7] Thus obesity raises basic social, economic, and political questions—for example, concerning urban planning and transport and food policy. Evidently, our current arrangements are fairly successful in many respects. Not only do they satisfy most basic needs, they also provide a range of pleasures and amenities appreciated by most members of Western societies. But both our food and transport systems are also costly and wasteful of energy and other scarce resources; they create significant environmental damage and pose a whole series of health risks, of which obesity is just one. Anyone who enjoys the benefits of supermarkets, fast and processed food, car travel, peaceful suburbs, and the like will be cautious about altering these systems. This caution remains justified even if one acknowledges that these goods also have significant costs and (as we stress in chapter 6) are sometimes matters of idealization or aspiration rather than straightforward reality. After all, it is no simple matter to say how we should alter such complex arrangements for the better, or who might assume the authority to do this.

But if there is not a single isolated problem, and since there are many layers of causation, we cannot expect there to be simple ways of reversing the rise of obesity, either in children or adults. To illustrate, consider the ambition of the United States' "Let's Move" campaign, spearheaded by Michelle Obama. This aims to "solv[e] the problem of obesity within a generation," primarily through the social marketing of physical activity and limited initiatives to improve access to healthy food.[8] Such a campaign may be well-intentioned and have

---

6. We mean this as a straightforwardly descriptive rather than derogatory term: under contemporary conditions, only an industrial food system can insure against widespread hunger.

7. But see Lee et al. (2002) for the interesting example of South Korea, which appears to have largely avoided significant obesity rates by retaining a traditional diet involving high rates of vegetable consumption. Its rates of obesity are increasing, however (OECD, 2012; Song et al., 2009).

8. "*Let's Move!* is a comprehensive initiative…dedicated to solving the problem of obesity within a generation, so that children born today will grow up healthier and able to pursue their dreams." See http://www.letsmove.gov/about, last accessed April 18, 2013.

helpful effects. But even if sustained for a generation, it will not "solve the problem of obesity," since it does not address the broader factors involved in Western diets and lifestyles. In those terms, even such a high-profile initiative can do little more than prompt some citizens to ask how greater rationality might be brought to bear on food production, transport, and built environments. Moreover, note that if Michelle Obama were to raise these questions herself, both she and her campaign would instantly be mired in party political polemics. Because food, transport, and planning systems are caught up with other freedoms and goods that people value—not to mention many vested and commercial interests—any attempt to alter them is bound to be controversial.

Thus responding to childhood obesity is a task that is fraught with difficulties, complexities, and uncertainties and raises many political questions. The simplest of these is the perennial question of priorities. What importance should we—be it as parents, citizens, or policy makers—attach to obesity prevention or reduction measures? How bold should we be in altering systems that, for all their risks and costs, also provide significant benefits? How should our societies combine their responses to this issue with responses to other urgent and deep-seated problems that they face? These are not questions that a book on childhood obesity can address. While we obviously believe that childhood obesity is a concern that deserves to be taken seriously, the question of how to tackle it alongside other priorities is ultimately one for democratic debate and decision.

As well as the question of priorities, issues of social concern—childhood obesity no less than any other—raise a second fundamental political question: how should responsibilities for action be divided between different actors? There are two slightly different things that we refer to in speaking of responsibilities for action. The most obvious concerns the need to take preventative or remedial action to address a societal problem: who has the duty or authority to do this? More fundamental still is the question of how we should be dividing basic social responsibilities. Are there principled ways to decide how to organize a society's "division of labor," or who should take responsibility for problems that emerge at a societal level? In speaking of a division of labor, we refer to the different roles that individuals and institutions play and how these are related to one another. In this way, a society can function as a cooperative endeavor and does not neglect important needs such as the well-being of its children. As we discuss in chapter 2, all societies assume that parents should play a large role here; but other institutions (such as schools and governments) also play a role, and other individuals are expected to play at least a minimal part (for example, in most societies parents can still assume that strangers will assist a child who is lost or distressed).

Again, the broad political principles governing such divisions of responsibility lie beyond our scope in this book. Given how central questions of social cooperation are for all matters of public policy, though, we believe it is worth emphasizing the degree of broad practical agreement that exists here. At first sight, disagreement about the role and responsibilities of the state, or indeed of companies and other institutions, may seem considerable. But there remains widespread agreement on at least two key points: First, governments must take some responsibility for public health. Second, where government policies affect people's health, they need to take account of those effects—especially if those policies are presently having a detrimental impact. All Western governments are extremely active in the fields of food and transport policy and urban planning. They spend a great deal of money on these things, and they support and regulate the various actors—both large companies and private individuals—in many ways. Plainly, this still leaves much room for disagreement and debate about the priority that health should take relative to other ends of policy, and the ways in which states can best regulate markets without damaging consumer freedoms and legitimate commercial interests. (In our context, those disagreements emerge most sharply with regard to taxation and marketing, considered in chapters 7 and 8.) But only ideologues who need take no responsibility for their positions claim that there is no role for government here.

Given the complexity of the problem, none of the possible interventions or policy measures promises immediate success in reducing rates of childhood obesity. Moreover, given these two much larger political questions—concerning priorities and the proper distribution of responsibilities—any proposed policy that does promise benefits in this dimension is likely to cause controversy because of its effects on other values and goals, or its implications for the responsibilities of different people and organizations. Although these factors deter us from offering straightforward prescriptions for action, we do not see them as reasons for pessimism, let alone inaction. In a complex situation, there will always be many opportunities for intervention, and we will try to highlight some of the most plausible modes of responding. Moreover, many of the possible measures can serve several goals and find support in our existing divisions of responsibility. For example, measures to address childhood obesity may also help to improve children's diets, educate them as independent consumers, increase their opportunities for physical activity, and so on. And they may be pursued through schools, as institutions that already have complementary responsibilities, or through regulatory frameworks that are already expected to take account of population health. In such ways, decisions among competing priorities can become much more tractable. There can be strong arguments for action even where definitive solutions are not available.

Summary of Individual Chapters

The book is divided into two parts. In the first part, we discuss some of the broader ethical issues posed by childhood obesity. In the second part, we turn to public policy issues by focusing on four different areas for intervention.

Part I. This section begins by considering the question of how much is known about childhood obesity and its effects, before turning to wider ethical questions about responsibilities to act and questions of justice and equality posed by childhood obesity.

Chapter 1. This chapter discusses the empirical data underlying the widespread concern with childhood obesity and emphasizes that this is more complex and uncertain than public discussions tend to acknowledge. Many claims made about health, diet, overweight, and obesity turn out to be difficult to substantiate in the bald terms in which they are often put forward. For example, there are difficulties in measuring obesity and in determining the health risks bound up with it, as well as disputes about the degree to which childhood obesity carries on into adulthood. Moreover, as most experts admit, it remains uncertain how to design interventions and policies that will successfully tackle childhood obesity. As a result, our "common-sense" intuitions may often be defeated by the unexpected complexity of the issues and the limitations of the evidence available. This lack of simplicity may seem discouraging in formulating positive responses. Nonetheless, we believe it is important to acknowledge the limits of existing knowledge. On the one hand, it helps to discourage simplistic and tokenistic responses of the "Something Must Be Done" and "Something Is Better Than Nothing" varieties. On the other, it encourages us to connect obesity to a wider range of problems and to remain open to new evidence about it.

Chapter 2. Here we turn from empirical uncertainty to normative uncertainty to develop an argument already briefly sketched in this introduction. By "normative uncertainty," we mean the wide range of reasonable disagreements that exist about what ought to be done—by individuals, organizations, or the state. We underline one of the main reasons for such disagreements. Each person values many different things and needs to find a way to combine and balance these in his or her life. Sometimes this involves difficult dilemmas and sacrifices, with no clear correct answer. More often, it is possible to find ways of combining these, but there may be different ways to do this too, and it may not be obvious which is best. In politics and in organizations, we often face similar problems in combining and balancing the different things that matter. One question for any reader of this book is how important childhood obesity is as an issue, and how our responses to it can fit alongside other priorities. At first sight, it may seem unhelpful to emphasize that we all have many goals, that priorities may be unclear and disputed, and that simple solutions are unavailable. We argue that this is not the case, however. Multiple goals and demands can often guide action much better than a single goal, especially (as stressed in chapter 1) when it is difficult to gain definitive information. This optimism is based on the fact that many options for intervening against childhood obesity might also fit with other desirable aims and goals. When this is true, policy makers do not need unambiguous evidence from scientific experts, since a policy that promises other benefits may well be worthwhile.

Chapter 3. Many debates about obesity raise the question of individual responsibility (Brownell et al., 2010; Kim & Willis, 2007). Arguments to the effect that people are responsible for their choices about eating and physical activity have been used to undermine claims that public funds should be used to address obesity, or that commercial food processing and marketing should be subject to regulation. Although fatter children are often bullied and blamed, public discussions do not endorse those attitudes. Instead, debates about childhood obesity tend to focus on parental responsibility. In this chapter, we look more closely at the difficult questions of causation and blame that are often raised concerning parents' roles, and argue that they point to a prior and more important question: what are the responsibilities that are properly borne by different people and organizations? No one doubts that parents must bear central responsibility for their children, but—despite the marked increase in rates of childhood obesity over recent decades—there is no reason to think that parents have started to take their responsibilities less seriously. As we discuss at greater length in chapter 6, what has changed is the environment that parents must navigate—for instance, the foods that are available and the way these are marketed to children. While debates often focus on the responsibility of parents, then, we argue that it is important to bear in mind how different people's and organizations' responsibilities interrelate and how a society's "division of labor" should be structured. We suggest that this provides a strong argument for revising the responsibilities of—among others—companies that manufacture and market processed foods, and that state regulation can actually be enabling for companies.

Chapter 4. In many industrialized countries, childhood obesity—like most other health problems—is more common among lower income and some ethnic minority groups. This raises concerns about equity. Policies that can successfully reduce childhood obesity among disadvantaged groups could make an important contribution to addressing social inequalities in health. However, experience in many health domains suggests that reaching these groups can be difficult, and it is not clear that low socioeconomic status groups will benefit from interventions to the same degree as better-off groups. We argue that it is important to consider the broadest possible range of effects that interventions and policies may have, and how these may be different for parents and families of different backgrounds. Sometimes, too, there may need to be trade-offs between health equality and other goals. For example, interventions may risk imposing additional burdens on low-income parents in order to achieve better health outcomes for their children. Likewise, tax policies (as considered further in chapter 7) may bite harder on lower-income families, but perhaps also confer greater benefits. We argue that such trade-offs need to be made explicit and carefully evaluated, not least by considering the views of those who will be affected by them.

Chapter 5. The final broad ethical issue that we consider is that of stigma. The discrimination and stigmatization that overweight and obese individuals face in Western societies is well documented, among children as well as adults. While media discussions sometimes suggest that stigmatization may motivate people to adopt healthier behaviors, research increasingly suggests that the opposite effect is more likely. In addition, the experience of stigma, teasing, and bullying clearly has significant and sometimes tragic costs for children's well-being. Moreover, social dislike of overweight is clearly related to widespread problems of unhealthy eating and unhealthy weight-loss strategies—problems that deserve attention alongside obesity prevention itself. (As we have pointed out already, childhood obesity is just one of many issues that merit social concern.) In this chapter, we argue that it is vital to consider and evaluate interventions and policies targeting childhood obesity to make sure that they do not have stigmatizing effects. We also argue that it is important to tackle weight-based stigma in its own right, since it is unjust and harmful to children.

Part II. Children and parents live in an environment that is shaped by many other people and organizations, and some of these other actors bear a clear responsibility for the rise in rates of obesity and lifestyle related ill-health.

Many policy initiatives have been based on individually oriented educational and informational measures. But it has also become clear that such measures rarely have significant effects if they are adopted on their own (Elinder, 2005; Lang & Rayner, 2007). In the second part of the book, we consider social and policy responses to this environment. We begin by discussing the social changes that have led commentators to speak of "obesogenic" environments, and then turn to three key areas for intervention: food pricing, food marketing, and the school system.

Chapter 6. The "obesogenic environment" is the focus of much debate about obesity's causes and possible responses to it. In this chapter, we first discuss what is meant by "obesogenic" and the wide range of different factors involved—such as transport infrastructures, food production and marketing systems, regulatory frameworks, and the cultures surrounding food and exercise. We then discuss the politics of making the "environment" a focus of concern. In particular, we argue that central features of our economies and societies may lead us to focus on individual choice and to ignore the complex systems on which our lives and choices depend. While the term "obesogenic environment" is sometimes criticized as vague, we suggest that it is helpful because it directs our attention to structural factors and the public responses they require. In the last part of the chapter, we consider some questions that arise when attempts are made to alter our environments. Structural policies generally have the advantages of affecting large numbers of people and not being seen to blame individuals for unhealthy behavior. However, as we discuss, they may be perceived as paternalistic; they may not always be equally beneficial to all, and in particular may make less of a difference than hoped to those who are already disadvantaged; and if targeted at particular groups (for instance, those of lower socioeconomic status), may be criticized as stigmatizing. While all these issues need consideration, we conclude that state and local government interventions to alter environments can be helpful and are called for.

Chapter 7. Proposals to alter food taxation and subsidy structures are now attracting public debate in many countries. Of particular relevance to children are high-profile proposals for a "soda tax," which have been especially controversial in the United States. Proposals to tax unhealthy foods are also being implemented in several European Union member states and promise especial impact on the situation of poorer families, who spend a higher proportion of their income on food. While tax policies obviously involve deliberate government interference in food prices, we argue that this is less of a departure than it might seem. Most Western states already interfere considerably in food markets. Apart from basic aspects of food safety, however, this is rarely with health-related aims in mind; for example, existing food subsidies tend to favor production of less healthy commodity foodstuffs and benefit large manufacturers of processed foods. Just like current policies, health-oriented tax and subsidy policies raise broader political questions about the limits and role of the state. However those questions are answered, we suggest that the proposals are valuable as a challenge or even a provocation. How can we address a situation where the cheapest foods tend to be high in calories, poor in other nutrients, and problematic for children's health?

Chapter 8. Alongside price, the marketing and availability of calorie-dense, nutrient-poor foods and drinks is of special concern for childhood obesity. Children are exposed to marketing through many channels, including television advertising, websites, food packaging that features familiar characters and celebrities, and the inclusion of free toys with food items. In this chapter, we ask what policies might address these influences. Different measures to restrict advertising have been employed in many countries, with varying stringency and success. In addition, counteradvertising, in the form of social marketing of health messages, has been widely attempted, although budgets are dwarfed by those of large companies. More recently, some attempts have been made to help children develop media literacy and understand the strategies and intentions behind advertising so that they are better able to resist its appeal. While each of these strategies may have only a limited effect on children's diets, we argue that they may complement one another and could be important planks in a broader strategy to address childhood obesity.

Chapter 9. In our final chapter, we explore the role that schools can play in tackling childhood obesity. Clearly, schools offer important opportunities to encourage healthier eating and physical activity habits in children. But some researchers have expressed disappointment at the limited effects of school-based interventions, while others argue that using schools to address wider social problems is tokenistic and interferes with schools' basic responsibilities. Building on one of our wider arguments, that interventions need to address a wide range of goals beyond childhood obesity, we consider how such interventions can fit within schools' existing responsibilities and complement other goals of the educational system. So long as they avoid harmful side effects (such as exacerbating stigma, for example), interventions targeting obesity and health can support schools' responsibility toward pupils' welfare and may assist in developing children's autonomy. The school setting also provides a promising opportunity to reach all children, regardless of socioeconomic background; however, much will depend on the design and distribution of interventions, and on whether they address the challenges of equity described in chapter 4. While there is potential for conflict between these kinds of interventions and schools' broader goals, we argue that well-designed interventions can avoid such conflicts and make a helpful contribution.

Conclusion

We began this introduction with some comments upon childhood and obesity as objects of concern. We would like to conclude it with a brief word about the other terms in this book's title: ethics and public policy. As should be clear already, we see these as closely related. Ethical questions primarily center on the actions and attitudes of individuals, while policy questions concern state action and the regulation of other actors, including individuals, schools, and companies. Evidently, the conduct of role-holders such as health professionals, teachers, or directors and employees of companies, sits somewhere in between: governmental and institutional policies shape their roles, while role-holders may also have responsibilities to implement, influence, and sometimes decide policies at different levels (see also Williams & Chadwick, 2012). More broadly, people's and organizations' responsibilities are shaped or affected by the responsibilities of those they interact with. For example, the responsibilities of parents are affected by the activities of food companies or schools or health organizations, or how far they may reasonably trust other adults to look out for their children. For these and other reasons, then, we will emphasize the interplay of ethical and policy issues.

From one perspective, this has the disadvantage of continually raising political questions. However, so long as these are approached with an openness to the many competing considerations involved, and without premature hopes of consensus on how to act, we see this as an advantage. After all, how a society brings up its children is bound to raise many questions of social cooperation and represents one of its most critical tasks. When a society's divisions of responsibility are widely accepted and successfully serve the many different goals that individuals and societies have, then it can enjoy the rare luxury of taking such arrangements for granted. Despite their relative stability and unprecedented prosperity, Western societies do not occupy such a fortunate position. Increasing rates of childhood obesity are just one of the problems that their public policy making must take account of. How to respond is inevitably a political question that concerns the balancing of many different goals and the proper allocation of responsibilities to many different actors.

As well as complementing on-going empirical research into the causes and effects of childhood obesity, then, we hope this book will complement discussions of other issues affecting children and health, including some that have been relatively neglected—for example, the dangers of widespread dieting and disordered eating, and the risks bound up with modern food production systems. In the end, no issue of public concern should be tackled without consideration of related concerns and competing priorities for action. While the resulting complexity may sometimes feel like a cause for dismay, it is also— as we will argue throughout—an important source of guidance. Policies to "solve the problem" of childhood obesity are not available. Nonetheless, there are many opportunities to address the issues involved, and many of the measures proposed to tackle childhood obesity promise other benefits too. Where we can find ways to act—whether individually or collectively—that constructively respond to many issues, it will be easier to foster agreement that meets the demands of ethics and politics alike.

MAJOR ETHICAL TOPICS

1

EMPIRICAL UNCERTAINTY

SOME DIFFICULTIES IN PLACING OBESITY CENTER STAGE

As we observed in the book's introduction, there is overwhelming evidence that the prevalence of childhood obesity has increased in most developed countries over the last twenty years (Ahrens et al., 2011b; Manios & Costarelli, 2011; Ogden et al., 2012). The importance of this rise lies in the range of conditions that are associated with obesity, including type 2 diabetes mellitus, fatty liver disease, endocrine and orthopedic disorders, and most of the major cardiovascular risk factors (Lobstein & Baur, 2005; Manios & Costarelli, 2011; Reilly et al., 2003), as well as the metabolic syndrome (Daniels et al., 2005; Steinberger et al., 2009; Weiss et al., 2004).

It is not a simple matter to interpret these facts and assess their significance, however. Especially in the media and in political debates, knowledge about obesity appears as more certain and less disputed than many experts would grant (Saguy & Almeling, 2008). Moreover, discussion often takes on a distinctly alarmist tone. The popular press has been full of references to an obesity "epidemic" (Flegal, 2006), an obesity "time bomb" (Doyle, 2003), or talk of parents who are "killing their children with kindness" (Martin, 2007). Drastic projections circulate about the current and future costs of treating the health effects of obesity and its costs in terms of economic productivity.[1] We are even warned that military capacity is suffering: "over 27 percent of all Americans 17 to 24 years of age—over nine million young men and women—are too heavy to join the military if they want to do so.... Being overweight is now by far the leading medical reason for rejection" (Mission: Readiness—Military Leaders for Kids, 2010, p. 2).[2] Perhaps the most memorable

---

1. We briefly consider these claims in chapter 2.

2. One might think this figure is already shocking enough, but it has even been turned on its head by some authors: "Because 75 percent of military applicants are

single claim started to circulate in the early 2000s, that the current generation would be the first to die sooner that its parents:

> Looking out the window, we see a threatening storm—obesity—that will, if unchecked, have a negative effect on life expectancy. Despite widespread knowledge about how to reduce the severity of the problem, observed trends in obesity continue to worsen. These trends threaten to diminish the health and life expectancy of current and future generations. (Olshansky et al., 2005, p. 1139)

This claim was quickly disputed (Couzin, 2005) and has yet to be substantiated (see Walls et al., 2012). Even one of the co-authors, David Allison, was soon quoted as saying, "These are just back-of-the-envelope, plausible scenarios. We never meant for them to be portrayed as precise" (in Gibbs, 2005, p. 73).

Other authors—"obesity critics," as we will refer to them—see such alarming claims as neither precise nor plausible. These critics dispute the idea that we are seeing a drastic increase in obesity that will have severe effects on population health. Instead of an "epidemic," they argue that we are seeing a relatively small shift in the average weight of the population (Campos et al., 2006). In addition, more recent data indicate that levels of obesity may have stopped increasing (e.g., Rokholm et al., 2010; Yanovski & Yanovski, 2011).

In this chapter, we emphasize some of the complexity and uncertainty surrounding childhood obesity, and how this permits wide divergences in opinion. A closer look often reveals limits to our knowledge—for example, with regard to such typical claims that the number of obese children continues to increase, that obese children will become obese and unhealthy adults, and that there are (or are not) effective interventions that can prevent childhood obesity. While it is beyond our scope to evaluate the evidence in each case, we believe it is important to appreciate the complexity of the issues and reasonable disagreements that exist here. None of this is to deny that obesity has significant health implications at the population level, nor is it to argue that

---

now rejected for obesity-related reasons, the past three US surgeons general and the chairman of the US Joint Chiefs of Staff have declared obesity a 'threat to national security'" (Lustig et al., 2012, p. 28); they cite no source, but the same figure appears in Daniel (2012). This in turn cites the Bipartisan Policy Center: Nutrition and Physical Activity Initiative (2012, p. 56), which accurately retails the figures from Mission: Readiness—Military Leaders for Kids (2010, p. 2).

nothing should be done because it is not clear what can be done. However, we do wish to emphasize that "the problem" itself is not as clear cut as it first appears, and that a myriad of possible relations and effects need to be borne in mind. Any clinician who deals with an obese child will be aware of this. His or her concern will never be directed only toward the child's obesity, and any practical measures or treatments will be intended to address a range of indications—invariably with the acknowledgment of many attending uncertainties in each regard. Policy makers cannot—for reasons we explore in the final section of chapter 2—be thought of as doctors tending the body politic, but a helpful parallel can still be drawn. Lacking complete knowledge of all the relevant causal pathways, so that it is impossible to pin down *the* problem (never mind how to "cure" it!), we must look to a broad range of evidence and acknowledge that there are many related aspects to be addressed (and no certainty of success!). We will develop this point in this and the next chapter, and argue that responses to childhood obesity need to engage not only with the many factors to which it appears to be related, but also with other social goals and priorities.

Causes, Complexity, and Uncertainty

Although the "cause" of obesity is often presented in simple terms, as an excess of energy intake compared to energy expenditure, obesity is far from simple. On the one hand, this shows up in the often-acknowledged difficulties of tackling obesity—whether at the level of individual treatment or of social prevention. On the other are the multitude of factors that have been associated with childhood obesity, and presumably stand in some causal relation to it. These include a whole raft of social factors: lower education levels (Lasserre et al., 2007; G. K. Singh et al., 2008; Sundquist & Winkleby, 2000), female gender (Matheson et al., 2008), belonging to racial or ethnic minorities (Ogden et al., 2010; Olshansky et al., 2005), and the built environment in which people live (Booth et al., 2005). Socioeconomic status has also been consistently linked with obesity levels (Robertson et al., 2007), and—as in the other cases just mentioned—there are probably several causal factors underlying this association.

In a now-famous attempt to summarize the causal complexity of obesity, the UK Foresight program mapped over a hundred relevant factors (Figure 1.1). But even this hugely complicated overview has significant omissions. Lack of sleep time has been consistently associated with childhood obesity and is

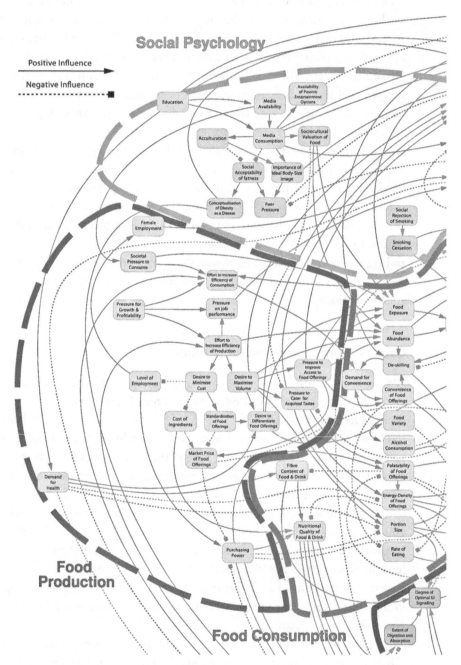

FIGURE 1.1 Close-up of the Foresight obesity system map, indicating some of the causal factors involved in obesity. For legibility, we reproduce only part of the diagram—factors relating to the physical activity environment and some physiological factors are not shown.

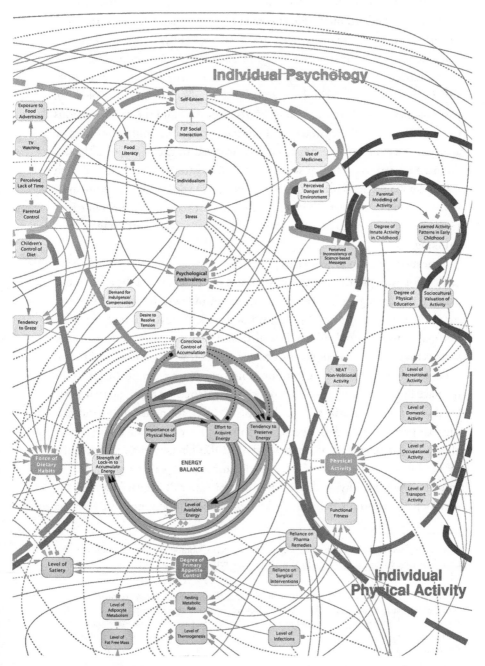

Source: Foresight (2007, p. 84f). Our reproduction omits color coding classifying the different causal factors. For the full diagram, please visit http://www.oup.com/us/voigt.

thought to play a causal role, but does not appear (Chen et al., 2008; Meyer et al., 2012). And although side effects of pharmaceutical drug use are mentioned (for instance, many women experience weight gain when taking the contraceptive pill), the role of obesogenic chemicals is also omitted.[3]

Moreover, this diagram only attempts to summarize the causes of obesity. One can imagine a similar exercise that would chart the physiological, psychological, social, and economic *effects* of obesity and the many relations that exist between these. In a slightly different way, one could also imagine a diagram setting out the causal factors involved in the forms of ill-health often associated with obesity, such as metabolic syndrome. The effect of such a diagram would be to place obesity—or better, the different factors involved in it—in a wider context. To imagine these and other possible diagrams is to raise the question as to how far obesity deserves to take center stage in our thinking.

The most prominent voices to pose this question are those of the obesity critics. For example, these authors may point out that many of the claims concerning the damaging health consequences of overweight and obesity rest on statistical associations. This means that weight or levels of body fat need not play a direct causal role in ill-health, and that we also need to consider factors that often occur alongside obesity. In other words, "overweight" and "obesity" may sometimes be confounding factors that should therefore be displaced from the center of our concern.[4] Evidence for thinking that body fat should not necessarily take pride of place can be found in studies indicating that persons classed as "overweight" do not necessarily have worse overall health outcomes (e.g. Carnethon et al., 2012; Uretsky et al., 2007; Calle et al., 2003).[5] Indeed, many overweight and obese persons appear to be "metabolically healthy"—that is, they do not suffer ill-health or any of the metabolic disruptions collectively known as metabolic syndrome (Ortega

---

3. As mentioned in the introduction to this book, the term "obesogen" refers to pollutants and chemicals that encourage obesity. In addition to the references given there, see Grün (2010) and Grün and Blumberg (2009).

4. All epidemiologists should be aware of the fallacies that can result from confusing association (or correlation) with causation. Association refers to any relationship between two factors, but this does not require a causal relationship. Over the past fifty years more people have started to wear jeans regularly, just as obesity rates have increased. This is a clear case of association *without* causation.

5. The term "obesity paradox" has been coined to refer to the protective effect of overweight against some disease, especially in older persons (Curtis et al., 2005; Chang et al., 2012; Ortega et al., 2013; cf. Walls et al., 2012). However, it has also been suggested that the apparent paradox could be the result of selection bias (Banack & Kaufman, 2013).

et al., 2013). Conversely, there are also studies of "metabolically obese but normal weight" individuals (Carnethon et al., 2012)—that is, persons who are not overweight but show evidence of poor metabolic health, sometimes including type 2 diabetes. More generally, the very complexity of the causal relations already suggests how difficult it is to demonstrate the exact importance of a single pathway. In particular, many of the factors involved—such as diet, physical activity levels, and environmental exposures—are extremely hard to measure objectively and hence more difficult to take account of in epidemiological studies. As elsewhere in life, our attention may be unduly captured by what is most readily seen and or most easily measured.

In the following sections we select some key uncertainties surrounding childhood obesity for closer inspection. First, we consider the measurement of childhood obesity through the application of the body mass index (BMI), as the commonest form of measurement used for obesity.[6] Second, we consider the association between childhood obesity and adult ill-health, since this is an association often invoked to justify early intervention. Third, we consider some problems in applying population-level generalizations at the individual level. Finally, we explore some uncertainties relating to the effectiveness of public health interventions. Each of these illustrates complexities inherent in childhood obesity, against the relatively simple claims that predominate in the media. As stated above, we do not regard these complexities as reasons for inaction. But we do regard them as reasons to think about obesity as one of *many* issues affecting children's current well-being and future health, and to be cautious in making it *the* central focus of attention.

Example 1: Obesity and the Application of the Body Mass Index

As something so fundamental to information about the problem of childhood obesity, one might hope that the definition of "obesity" itself would be beyond reproach. But upon closer examination definitions of obesity are subject to considerable variation. Likewise, there are significant problems in capturing obesity in terms of body mass index, despite its near-universal use.

Early definitions could be quite vague. Jutel notes that some authors referred to overweight in terms of physical bulk, using a social standard

---

6. For an extended discussion of the standardization and classification of the BMI, see Nicholls (2013).

of what was deemed "sightly" as the threshold for determining overweight (Jutel, 2006). Subsequently, overweight was defined in terms of body *mass*, or relative *weight*, as distinguished from obesity as a condition characterized by excessive body *fat* (Himes & Dietz, 1994). On current definitions, however, both overweight and obesity are seen as indices of body fat. This is generally based on the assumption that health risks materialize as excess body fat increases:

> Ideally, health-oriented definitions of overweight *and* obesity should be used that are based on the amount of excess body fat at which health risks to individuals increase. (Hubbard, 2000, p. 1067, emphasis added)

Since the general adoption of the BMI, there has also been a gradual move toward a universal standard of categories for overweight and obesity (Ebbeling & Ludwig, 2008). Thus, prior to 1999, many experts considered a BMI of 29 kg/m² to be overweight. Later this was reduced to 27 kg/m² and today a BMI above 25 kg/m² is the standard used to indicate overweight in adults (Ross, 2005). This gradual reduction and standardization of categories simplifies and, at least for nonexperts, may make matters appear more settled than they in fact are.

However, remaining definitional questions can mean that the same terminology refers to manifestly different entities, since body fat and body weight are not tightly related. If obesity is defined in terms of the amount of adipose tissue, this requires a method of assessment that gauges body fat percentage, such as underwater weighing or tricep skinfold thickness. These methods require more time, expense, and expertise than a simple weighing scale. Studies comparing body fat percentage with BMI have found that the number of "obese" participants differs enormously depending on which measure is used (Flegal, 1993; Ortega et al., 2013). Flegal, for example, recounts two studies (Gortmaker et al., 1987; Harlan et al., 1988) that used the same data set and yet came to diametrically opposite conclusions regarding trends in obesity prevalence. On Flegal's analysis, the conclusions depended precisely on the measures used.[7] The underlying problem is that while BMI is (partly) correlated with percentage of body fat (Smalley et al., 1990;

---

7. In addition, many studies rely on individuals' or parents' reports of weight and height, rather than measuring these directly. This introduces not only inaccuracy (since many people do not know or report these accurately) but also systematic bias (since people tend to under-report weight, and do so to a greater degree as weight increases) (Yanovski & Yanovski, 2011).

Widhalm et al., 2001), it is also correlated with bone density and mass more generally. Notoriously, muscular athletes may therefore be classed as overweight or even obese in terms of BMI.

In addition, assessment of fat mass—difficult to perform on large numbers of people—hardly reveals the full story. The body can store fat in different locations, and it has long been observed that the distribution of adipose tissue is important in health terms. Abdominal (or "visceral") fat that appears around the waist is associated with worse health, while fat stored beneath the skin ("subcutaneous"), for instance on the hips and thighs, is not. (This is the colloquial difference between "apple" and "pear"-shaped bodies. See Bazzocchi et al., 2012.) While adiposity is more precise than BMI, then, it still obscures physiological differences that have significant implications for metabolism and health.

In the case of children, the issue is even more complicated because the proportion and distribution of fat on the body naturally alters with development and growth, just as bone and muscle mass do. Because of this additional complexity, growth charts are used to compare children against others of the same age and sex. Thus the standard approach is now to use reference centiles. A child whose BMI lies on the 80th centile, for example, has a BMI that is greater than that of 80 percent of other children of the same age and sex. To assess an individual in this way thus requires the prior selection and measurement of a reference cohort in order to discover a "standard" range and distribution of BMI. In addition, demarcations—or "cut points"—must be selected to classify children as, for example, "underweight" or "overweight." In the United States the 85th centile has been used to define overweight, and the 95th obese. In a UK-based reference population, alternatives such as the 91st, 97.7th, and 99.6th centiles have been used (Power et al., 1997). Ideally, these boundaries would relate to health risks, yet in practice

> such a point cannot be identified with any precision, for three reasons: (a) children have less obesity-related disease than adults, (b) the link between child obesity and adult health risk is mediated through adult obesity and adult disease, and (c) the dose-response curve linking obesity and outcome is essentially linear over a broad spectrum of adiposity, so that no obvious cut-off point exists. This makes the setting of a cut-off essentially arbitrary. (Cole & Rolland-Cachera, 2002, p. 15)

The selection of 85th and 95th centiles was made in order to correspond with adult BMI categories at age 18 (Cole et al., 2000). Apart from questions about whether this is really the age at which people should be considered biologically mature (see also Reilly, 2006, p. 596), it should be appreciated that in children these points have no clinical basis, and have simply been chosen to mesh with adult categories.

As this suggests, assessments of childhood obesity have followed the attempts at standardization seen in adults. Reference growth curves are now derived from pooled international data sets in order to create international standards. For example, the widely used International Obesity Task Force (IOTF) standards are based on six nationally representative cross-sectional surveys of children's growth from Brazil, Great Britain, Hong Kong, the Netherlands, Singapore, and the United States. In part, this has been a response to the varying percentiles selected in different studies and guidelines, aiming at standardization and reduction of variation between studies (and the corresponding uncertainty this variation generates) (Cole et al., 2000; Himes & Dietz, 1994). However, this may generate the misleading impression that standards are applicable irrespective of context and involve assumptions that may not hold for populations that were not part of the original reference data. Perversely, if populations are sufficiently heterogeneous, then pooling data may generate a reference standard that is not applicable to any particular population because it averages out variations between populations living in differing circumstances or perhaps with different genetic characteristics. Hence, it may be that effects specific to particular populations are missed (again, see Reilly, 2006), and there remains on-going debate regarding national and international reference standards (Must & Anderson, 2006).

These varying standards can have a substantial impact. This is nicely demonstrated in a study of overweight and obesity in Czech seven-year-old children (Kunešová et al., 2011). The study compared reference standards from the World Health Organization (WHO) and the IOTF, as well as Czech national standards. When applied to the same data, Czech and IOTF values indicated that the combined prevalence of overweight and obesity in boys was 14.8 percent and 15.8 percent respectively. By contrast, the WHO cut-offs suggested the combined prevalence in boys was 23.5 percent. While it is no surprise that the definition of categories has a significant impact on the results obtained, such large variations are plainly troubling. It is still possible, of course, to gauge changes in BMI within populations using one or the other categorization, but the different categories may have important and misleading consequences for our perception of the situation and the need for intervention.

Example 2: Childhood Obesity and Its Relation to Adult Ill-Health

To what extent does obesity at a particular stage of childhood predict—or as it is sometimes put, "track"—obesity or ill-health in adulthood? This question is especially important when we consider the priority that should be given to policies aimed at obesity prevention or treatment in children. A failure of obesity to track from childhood into adulthood would indicate that policies that focus on treating obese children are less important and that broader preventive policies would most likely be preferable. Indeed, policies that target obese children could create needless concern or have other harmful effects (Szwarc, 2004).

There are several important questions about how to frame the issues that have attracted rather different responses and that give rise to differing results. As already reported, how obesity and overweight are used and defined varies between studies (Reilly et al., 2003). Moreover, definitions of childhood also differ. In a review by Reilly et al., an inclusion criterion of ages 1–18 was used, whereas a systematic review by Singh et al. considered childhood to be ≤12 years, and adolescence to be ≥13 years but ≤18 years (A. S. Singh, et al., 2008). In addition, findings depend on the modes of measurement used and the variables taken into account. In their systematic review, Singh et al. note that there is a stronger tracking of childhood obesity into adulthood when BMI rather than skinfold thickness is used (A. S. Singh et al., 2008). In addition, there may be further determinants that are only considered in some studies. For example, some models include parental weight while others do not. The inclusion of parental weight is reported to increase the predictive power of childhood obesity trends (Robertson et al., 2007) and its omission may therefore be significant.

The data on tracking also reflects the subjective nature of interpretation through terms such as "good," "poor," or "adequate." In one analysis, Wright and colleagues suggest that correlation coefficients of $r = 0.24$ and $r = 0.39$ indicate that "body mass index in childhood showed a moderate, significant correlation with adult body mass index" (Wright et al., 2001, p. 1281).[8] In

---

8. The correlation coefficient, represented by the letter r, indicates the strength of a relationship between two variables, on the assumption that this relationship is linear. A value of 1 indicates a perfect proportionality between the two variables, while a value of 0 indicates that there is no (linear) relationship. (If $r = 0$, this does not mean that there is no relationship—for example, visual analysis may show a significant nonlinear relationship: when age and mortality are compared, a U-shaped curve is seen, corresponding to high levels of mortality in early childhood, reducing levels in childhood and early adulthood and increasing levels at older age.)

a separate paper, a similar correlation coefficient of $r \approx 0.30$ is described as "moderate to poor" (Power et al., 1997, p. 511), while in their analysis within the Bogalusa Heart Study, Freedman et al. describe a correlation of childhood and adult BMI of $r = 0.6$ as "moderate" (Freedman et al., 2009, p. 753), despite using the term "moderate" to refer to $r = 0.33–0.41$ in a previous study (Freedman et al., 2005, p. 25).

Moreover, the perspective applied to the data can affect one's interpretation. Hesketh et al. (2003), for example, report that 19.8 percent of those children classified as overweight or obese at baseline were no longer so three years later. Similarly, Whitaker et al. (1997) report that 83 percent of 10- to 14-year-olds with a BMI above the 95th percentile were obese as adults. Both studies judge that there is a strong tracking of childhood obesity to adulthood. Yet Voss et al. cite these findings—that almost 20 percent of obese 5- to 10-year-olds had spontaneously resolved to a healthy weight within three years—as evidence that BMI tracks relatively poorly from early childhood to adulthood (Voss et al., 2006). Instead of asking how many obese children become obese adults, we may ask what percentage of obese adults were also obese children. One study found that while 83 percent of overweight or obese youth were overweight or obese as adults, 85 percent of overweight or obese adults were classed as normal weight in their youth (Herman et al., 2009). Presenting the data in this manner suggests a much weaker relationship between child and adult obesity.

These examples demonstrate that even when numerical data are available and the classificatory boundaries are accepted, their interpretation and integration with other knowledge is far from straightforward and may generate quite different assessments. A focus on the tracking of childhood obesity into adulthood may lead to the conclusion that prevention should be targeted toward obese children. In contrast, if our attention is on those adults who are obese then more general population measures may be deemed appropriate, given the large percentage of normal weight children who become overweight or obese adults.[9]

Example 3: The Individualization of BMI

In general, classification collates items in order to facilitate tasks such as counting or comparing (Bowker & Starr, 1999). In the context of healthcare we may

---

9. For additional recent review of the evidence here, see Park et al. (2012).

want to know how many people are sick in order to inform treatment protocols, health service planning, or budgeting (Jutel, 2009). One of the consequences of classification, however, is that grouped items tend to be perceived as more similar than items that exist outside of the class—something that poses problems when the traits in question are continuous (as measurements on a numerical scale are). The *intra*class differences are downplayed, while the *inter*class differences are exaggerated (Tajfel, 1981; Zerubavel, 1996). Using the example of boxing weight categories, Zerubavel (1996) notes: "we perceive the metrically negligible "distances" between 119-pound ("bantamweight") and 120-pound ("featherweight") boxers…as greater than those between 120-pound and 125-pound (both "featherweight") boxers" (p. 425). Similarly, the classification of individuals as normal weight, overweight, or obese diminishes the differences that exist *within* weight categories while at the same time increasing perceptions of differences *between* classes. For example, the difference between normal weight and overweight is potentially the difference between a BMI of 24.9 and 25.0, while the within group variation of normal weight can be as much as the difference between a BMI of 18.0 and 24.9.

Underlying this problem is a deeper one, that selecting out one dimension for comparison necessarily pushes the many other possible dimensions of comparison away from center stage. In boxing, this may not be problematic—apart from weight, only one other dimension of comparison is relevant, and that is precisely the fighting ability that is tested in the ring. But when one thinks of human health, there is a near-infinity of such factors—many hardly reducible to a linear scale—that may be relevant. (Consider again the Foresight obesity diagram, above, for a small selection of these.)

This simple fact gives rise to enormous problems if population-level measures are applied to individuals. Tajfel (1981) refers to this as "personalization":

> If there is to be an explanation in terms of the characteristics of a group, these must be characteristics which are relevant to the situation and *common* to the whole group, with a corresponding neglect of individual differences between the members of a group. (p. 138)

In turn, this can lead to the assumption that health effects found at the *group* level—for example, the group of obese persons—must be shared by the *individuals* within the group—for example, those classed as obese by their individual BMI. This ignores the variation within this classification, including a vast range of respects in which each individual differs from other people placed in the same category.

As BMI has gained currency, it has become much more common to use it in screening and clinical applications. BMI was originally conceived as "Quetelet's index" in the 1800s (Smalley et al., 1990). This index was devised after plotting a range of heights and weights of army conscripts (Oliver, 2006), whereby Quetelet noted a Gaussian distribution of the population—the familiar bell-shaped curve that statisticians call "normal." This allowed the description of the (statistically) average man, as well as the use of statistical techniques to determine (statistically) significant deviations from the norm (Oliver, 2006). But this exercise was merely descriptive and obviously restricted to a specific subgroup of the population.

Yet the technique remained and was later employed in a health-related context with the use of actuarial "build cards" that were used to develop risk policies based on actual and expected deaths of policy owners. The tables derived the weight-for-height associated with minimal mortality among policy holders (Jutel, 2009). Again, this was a population-level analysis—consistent with epidemiological methods that assess aggregate data at the population level—although it was again based on a restricted population (that is, the owners of life assurance).

More recently the IOTF has developed half-year cut-offs for children between 2 and 18 years of age. In their recent survey of methodological aspects of childhood obesity epidemiology, Rodríguez et al. (2011) note that these standards should only be used to assess overweight prevalence at the population level, since the standards "do not have enough accuracy and precision at the individual level" (p. 24). For the same reason, many have cautioned that BMI should not be used diagnostically (Kuczmarski & Flegal, 2000), and that definitions of overweight using BMI, while valuable for general public health surveillance, screening, and similar purposes, "do not necessarily identify physiological states per se" (Flegal et al., 2006, p. 757). As stressed above, the centile equivalents in children and adolescents were derived in order to make comparisons between populations and to assess trends, not for the purpose of individual diagnosis. In other words, BMI categories were designed for use at the population level, and *not* for clinical assessment of individuals.

Despite these cautions, the IOTF cut-offs for pediatric "overweight" and "obesity" are often used in the clinic (Voss et al., 2006) and, as we discuss in chapter 2, in school-based measuring programs. For example, materials from the UK's National Child Measurement Program tell parents that "you can receive your child's individual results. This will help you to know if your child is in the healthy weight range. If your child is overweight, further support is available from your local NHS" (NHS Choices, 2010). This reference to the National Health Service implies that overweight status is inherently problematic in health terms. Yet BMI categorization represents an extremely simplistic assessment, and—as we stress in chapter 2 when discussing such measuring programs—pays no attention to the general health of the child.

This is not an isolated example. The Australian National Health and Medical Research Council (NMHRC) explicitly states that "BMI-for-age percentile charts *should be used in clinical practice*...a BMI above the 85th percentile being indicative of overweight and a BMI above the 95th percentile being indicative of obesity" (National Health and Medical Research Council [Australia], 2003, p. 14, emphasis added). This flatly contradicts earlier cautions that BMI should not be used diagnostically. Using BMI cut-offs to assess individuals simplifies the relationship between overweight or obesity and health implications for the individual. It does so because it ignores individual differences in relative muscle, bone-mass, and fat tissue distribution and—still more important—fails to take account of other determinants and aspects of health. As Ross (2005) notes, "the 'risk' referred to in epidemiological studies of obesity is the *prevalence of a given disease in populations* of people...not the personal risk that a person...has of getting that disease" (p. 100, emphasis added). The application of population-derived risk estimates to individuals increases the danger of inappropriate clinical intervention, not to mention the anxiety that parents are likely to feel and the worry and stigma that a child may experience.

We do not say this in order to advise clinicians how to do their job. Clinical judgment naturally considers a variety of criteria and indications and draws on many sources of evidence. Our point is only that BMI—let alone the broader classifications of "overweight" and "obese"—has grave limitations. Above all, these should caution nonexperts from making judgments upon such a basis. Most parents, we suspect, are very well aware of this and would naturally resist judgments that their child urgently requires intervention simply on the basis of a relatively high BMI (for his or her age and sex), without attention to a whole range of other factors. As we will argue throughout this book, a parallel point applies at the population level, too. That is to say, in judging what sorts of intervention and policy are appropriate, we will need to take account of much more than obesity levels or obesity prevention.

Example 4: Uncertainty in the Effects of Public Health Interventions

The first two uncertainties considered above make judgments about health and health policy much more difficult, while the third problem concerns the caution necessary when applying findings to individuals. Finally, we briefly consider another area of difficulty concerning the evidence base for policy interventions designed to prevent obesity or reduce its incidence. (On the parallel difficulties concerning measures to help individual children who are already overweight or obese, or to prevent an individual child becoming obese, see Hammer [2010].)

The difficulty of assessing childhood obesity interventions is considerable; the result is that the literature contains significant disagreements and many unresolved questions. This is not for want of attempts to review and synthesize the large amount of research that has been done—there are many systematic reviews relating to obesity-related outcomes, diet, physical activity levels, and more. The problem is rather the enormous number of variables in play. This creates immense difficulties in precisely documenting interventions and comparing them against one another. Interventions tend to involve many different elements conducted in rather different social, political, and organizational settings. In addition, interventions tend to have multiple aims, and—since obesity is, as we will continue to stress, not a simple target so far as health is concerned—these aims need not be primarily focused on obesity levels.[10] (They might focus, less ambitiously, on changing dietary, sleep, or sedentary behaviors; it is also conceivable that they might, more ambitiously, focus on health outcomes.) This also creates significant problems in assessing the effectiveness of different interventions, since the criteria of assessment cannot meaningfully be reduced to a single one—for example, whether there was a reduction in average age-adjusted BMI levels. All of these difficulties are compounded by the well-known problems of publication bias—for understandable (if not defensible) reasons, ineffective interventions are less likely to be written up or be accepted for publication. The same point also applies at a more subtle level: the lack of effectiveness of an intervention on a particular dimension is less likely to attract published comment, as compared with discussion of its more effective elements.

These issues are highlighted in an important discussion article by Doak et al. (2009). This considers two independent reviews of interventions to prevent obesity that were conducted by different co-authors of the subsequent

---

10. As the authors of a nice discussion of multiple reviews regarding the effectiveness of community interventions to promote physical activity comment: "There was an inevitable tension in this analysis between a narrowness that ensured that all reviews were on exactly the same topic, and a breadth that ensured all potentially relevant reviews were included; the same tension concerning homogeneity of focus as exists in many systematic reviews in public health" (Woodman et al., 2012, p. 17). See also another recent review by Metcalf et al. (2012).

discussion. The earliest review (Doak et al., 2006) implicitly noted the effect of framing on the outcome of the review in considering previous reviews and their limitations. It also noted much variation in outcome measures and suggested that this prevents the meta-analysis of results. Despite these difficulties, the authors concluded that 17/25 (68 percent) of the studies identified should be considered effective. However, a Cochrane review, which included 22 interventions, suggested that only four of these were effective (18 percent) (Summerbell et al., 2005). The authors of the latter review conclude, in direct contrast to Doak et al., that "the interventions employed to date have, largely, not impacted on weight status of children to any significant degree" (Summerbell et al., 2005, p. 37).

Such conflicting findings are evidently perplexing, and the welcome result was a discussion piece jointly written by both sets of authors. In it, they note that only 10 studies appeared in both articles, a clear example of the effect that differing criteria for inclusion have on the outcome of a research review. In each case, there were plausible reasons for inclusion and exclusion—this was not a problem of arbitrariness, and the subsequent discussion shows that the differing criteria applied could be justified, even where there is subsequent agreement that one decision was better than another. For example, all authors endorse the decision to exclude studies of shorter duration, and indeed argue that a minimum study length should be six months. However, it is possible that short interventions could have effects, and this might be very welcome from a policy perspective. The authors of the Doak review also tracked down unpublished data so that they could fully compare outcomes of the studies. While the subsequent consensus was that such data should not be admitted, since it has not been subject to peer review, it is easy to see how one might reach the opposite conclusion. The results that researchers omit are likely to reflect the publication bias mentioned above; including only published data may create a false appearance of greater effectiveness.

As well as different opinions as to whether a study should be included in a review, the reviews also used different criteria to gauge effectiveness. While both focused on weight outcomes only, they took different views on the assessment of studies where the outcomes did not all point in the same direction—as is often the case:

> Where discordant outcomes were reported, Summerbell et al. decided on effectiveness using mean change in BMI. The Doak et al. review accepted any statistically significant, beneficial change in

anthropometric outcomes as evidence of an "effective" intervention, even where there were discordant results. Discordant assessment of outcomes explains differences in the classification of three articles as effective [by Doak et al.] versus not effective. These differences relate to results that were not [classified as] effective by the Summerbell et al. review because they were not effective by mean BMI change, but were effective by other measures, such as prevalence change, effect on slope of BMI in a multivariate model for girls or an effective result for skin-folds. (Doak et al., 2009, p. 353)

As one might expect, then, findings depended on the outcomes sought. What a pragmatically minded reader might not expect, however, is that it is no simple matter to judge what counts as effectiveness or how it should be measured. Indeed, this was one point on which the review authors reached no consensus. In sum, "the totality of evidence can look very different depending on how the systematic review is designed. The question remains, what are the appropriate criteria to apply?" (Doak et al., 2009, p. 353).

Note, moreover, that further uncertainties arise since interventions may have had—or failed to have—additional effects that were not only excluded from the review, but also from consideration within the original studies. A focus only on reduction in average BMI (or percentage of body fat) or the number of children classified as obese is just one indicator of health-related outcomes, and perhaps not the most significant in the longer-term, especially so far as wider health effects are concerned. The difficulty for anyone designing and evaluating an intervention is that the potential criteria involved here are enormously wide and include many factors that are extremely difficult to measure objectively (such as long-term changes in dietary habits) or whose importance depends on explicitly moral and political judgment (for example, one might ask how far participants found the intervention to be worthwhile or effective on their own terms). Or as Hillier et al. (2011) comment, in discussing the evidence base for childhood obesity prevention, "from the child's perspective it is the psychosocial consequences of being overweight or obese rather than the health issues which are more important" (p. 259). (We will return to the difficult question of judging which effects should be of greatest priority in chapter 2.) The result is that a question that sounds very simple—"What works?"—turns out to be difficult to decide and involves many complex and disputable questions of judgment.

Conclusion

In this opening chapter we have considered some empirical uncertainties presented by research on childhood obesity. Uncertainties exist as to the very definition of obesity, its relation to adult health and weight, the ways in which BMI is relevant to individuals, and how to gauge the effects of interventions meant to address obesity. There are many other examples we could have considered. Debates continue, for example, as to how important changes in diet are in causing rising levels of obesity compared to changes in levels of physical activity—not to mention a host of other factors such as too little sleep or chemicals used in food processing and household objects. Do particular nutrients—fats, simple carbohydrates, caloric sweeteners in drinks—play a greater role than other sources of calories? How far does the stigma and prejudice that fatter children face itself contribute to ill-health? The list could continue, and should suggest a wider point. Uncertainties may often be increased rather than diminished by the research process, as we come to appreciate the number of interacting factors and possible causal pathways.[11]

Of course, to emphasize all this uncertainty may seem unhelpful. For example, how is policymaking to respond when scientists disagree about the definition of "the problem" and how to address it? Nonetheless, we believe that a little modesty about the limits of our knowledge represents a much-needed caution. Critics of the recent emphasis on obesity can make strong arguments that alarmist claims have led to unproven—and potentially ineffective or damaging—interventions, both for individuals and at the policy level (see also Gard, 2011a). If "Something Must Be Done" then too often it seems that "Something (Anything!) Is Better Than Nothing." Needless to say, that is not a logical entailment.

At the same time, to emphasize the uncertainties may give rise to a rather different refrain: "more research is needed." Anyone who is curious about the world can agree with this injunction. Nonetheless, we should also be aware of how often it has been misused. The tobacco industry made great play of it, and manufacturers of processed foods and drinks have found it just as useful in the obesity context. A need for more research does not entail that there is no need for action, and this is certainly not what we intend to argue. While we have not emphasized this side of the story, none of the uncertainties we are

---

11. This may seem somewhat pessimistic, and we do not deny that further research may clarify issues. Our point is only that more empirical data does not always resolve existing uncertainty and may instead reveal further layers of complexity or new interpretative possibilities.

aware of undercuts the substantial evidence indicating that children have, on average, become fatter, and that this is, on average, bound up with risks and costs to present and future health. But the many difficulties involved in defining the exact problem, or the measures that would undo it, strongly argue against the sort of "tunnel vision" that situates obesity at the center of our attention. No clinician or parent would permit this in dealing with an individual child, nor should we be tempted by it at the policy level. Rather, we need to situate obesity alongside other related factors that affect large numbers of children—such as low levels of physical fitness and high levels of fat and sugar consumption, not to mention a host of other factors, such as high levels of disordered eating, stigma, and discrimination—and think about how best we can respond to these together. Or so we will argue in chapter 2.

2 NORMATIVE UNCERTAINTY

WHAT DO WE WANT FROM POLICIES TO ADDRESS CHILDHOOD OBESITY?

In chapter 1 we considered some of the difficult issues surrounding empirical claims and evidence in debates about childhood obesity. Our "common-sense" judgments may often be defeated by the unexpected complexity of the issues and the limitations of the evidence available. Even in scientific and policy discussions, many common claims about health, diet, overweight, and obesity turn out to be difficult to substantiate, at least in bald or straightforward terms.

In this chapter, we suggest that the issues are also less straightforward than they may appear when we turn our attention to *normative* questions—that is, questions about what ought to be done. The question "What do we want from policies to address childhood obesity?" is deliberately provocative. In one sense, the answer is so obvious as to need no stating: we want to prevent obesity.[1] But this answer is radically unsatisfactory in three key respects. First, merely to state this goal leaves open the question: *why* do we want to prevent obesity? Perhaps the answers we give to this question may suggest that obesity prevention should not always be our first consideration or explicit priority. For example, if improved health and longevity is the underlying motivation for obesity prevention policies, then other goals may be more important. Second, we may not be in a good position to judge whether we are achieving this goal. Some of the empirical uncertainties considered in the last chapter point to difficulties in assessing whether a policy measure has succeeded in reducing obesity rates, let alone in improving health. Third, public policy seeks to achieve many things, of which reduced obesity rates and improved health are only two examples.

---

1. Later in this chapter, we briefly discuss issues of prevention versus treatment. Since our concern is with children's situation, however, prevention obviously takes first place.

Policies that aim at these particular goals will also have wider effects as well as opportunity costs. Notoriously, other policies—be they economic or social or industrial—often have effects on health outcomes or obesity rates too.

At first glance, it may seem unhelpful to underline these complexities. Just like an emphasis on how complex and uncertain the evidence is, an emphasis on how complex and contested our goals are may seem to paralyze action. As one author put it, referring to the Foresight report's (in)famous obesity system map (2007, p. 84f, see figure 1.1, this volume):

> the danger of wrapping an issue such as obesity up in the language of sociology and systems analysis is that it all begins to seem impossibly complicated. It is as if one needs to solve all the problems of society to tackle one relatively small sub-problem. So the government's strategy includes food supply, education, the design of towns, primary care, walking kids to school, tackling false perceptions, counseling, old Uncle Tom Cobley and all. (Hawkes, 2008, p. 1204)

Such impatience is readily understandable—life would be much simpler if it weren't so darned complicated. Unfortunately, the fact remains that most problems facing public policy do not come neatly defined, ready to be picked off one-by-one with a silver bullet. Rather, as Rittel and Webber (1973) famously put it, they tend to be "wicked problems"—bound up in complex systems, where different people and organizations have different perspectives, and where the interventions made by different actors are rarely predictable or measurable in their effects, and often have unwanted side effects. So there are neither discrete, unambiguous problems nor simple, straightforward solutions.

Fortunately, we do not have to sacrifice realism and maturity in order to act in the face of complexity—or so we will argue in this chapter. Not only is this problem a complex one; it is also true that the aims of public policy are themselves multiple and complex. We see this as a cause for optimism rather than despair, because multiple goals can often guide action much better than a single one, especially when it is difficult to achieve comprehensive and definitive information. Our optimism here—and throughout this book— is based on the fact that many options for intervening to tackle childhood obesity might also fit with other desirable aims and goals (Robinson, 2010; Swinburn, 2008; see also Foresight, 2007, p. 124ff). When this is the case, we do not need unambiguous evidence of effectiveness, neither before nor following a policy measure. This is not to say that evidence doesn't matter; but we need to look to many sources of evidence and a variety of goals, and accept that evaluation is rarely straightforward.

This chapter proceeds as follows. First, it considers the proper rationale for obesity prevention policies. We argue that this should be squarely focused on the health and well-being of those who might suffer obesity-related ill-health. Second, we argue that health promotion is itself a complex goal, which is surrounded by many other proper goals of public policy. However, multiple goals are ubiquitous and (in general) helpful for decision making. We suggest that this fact poses problems for "single-issue" policies. As examples, we briefly consider informational campaigns designed to promote healthier behavior and programs to measure children's BMI. Given the many goals people and policies must pursue, we argue that there are good reasons to expect such closely targeted policies to be relatively ineffective and even to have unfortunate side effects. We conclude the chapter by discussing how action is possible in the face of both empirical and normative uncertainty.

Why Should We Seek to Prevent Childhood Obesity?

Preventing childhood obesity is not an end in itself. Instead, we contend that the principal rationale for prevention policies is, and can only be, the health of the persons involved. In particular, we argue that neither social prejudice against fatter people nor the projected costs of treating the ill-health of fatter people constitute defensible grounds for obesity prevention policies.

"Fat-ism"

As we discuss in chapter 5, many social prejudices in Western societies incline people to dislike fat bodies. However, few people would explicitly endorse these feelings as a rationale for any public policy, or as a basis for encouraging others to lose weight or stay slim. But when we think about children's lives, perhaps these claims may seem too quick. One might argue that given such social prejudices, overweight and obese children are disadvantaged and likely to suffer many ill-effects, independently of any physiological relation between fatness and ill-health; and this gives good grounds to take preventative or remedial action. This suggestion is more problematic than it might seem, however. It is certainly true that parents—if not policy makers—legitimately take an interest in a child's future appearance and perhaps even attractiveness.

However, there is considerable evidence that a preoccupation with body weight is damaging to children's development: it is a well-known factor in the development of eating disorders; more generally it tends to damage children's self-conception, body image, and attitudes to food (Goldschmidt et al., 2010; Raudenbush & Bryk, 2002; Wong et al., 2011).

More broadly, there are familiar difficulties with recommendations based on recognized social prejudices—in this case, widely shared aesthetic and sexual preferences for slimmer bodies, which diminish the social status of fatter people in many ways. As a comparison, consider the use of skin-lightening creams in a racist society. Already stigmatized individuals may have little power to challenge racist attitudes; depending on the case, their best course of action may be to do what they can to avoid being the subject of such prejudice—for example, to "pass" (as white), as it used to be said. Parents may feel equally powerless as regards their children, but here the dilemmas may seem even more uncomfortable: to help a child be white(r) or thin(ner) involves educating him or her in the social condemnation. Indeed, as we will argue in the following chapters, this stigma makes it much more difficult for parents to respond when their child is becoming overweight or obese, because no parent wants to convey to a child that there is anything wrong with his or her body or appearance.

This is the situation of individuals who face a society that thinks and acts in a prejudiced, stigmatizing way. Public policy must consider how institutions should respond on behalf of society as a whole. Of course, widely shared prejudice makes it more difficult to respond appropriately. Nonetheless, from this perspective, the most direct and obvious recommendation is to challenge the prejudice itself. At the very least, we must be wary of rationalizing obesity prevention policies in terms of the psychosocial harms or social disadvantages that overweight and obese individuals may experience. That such harms and disadvantages exist is clear. If all overweight and obesity were prevented, then perhaps no one would experience those harms and disadvantages.[2] But their cause is not overweight or obesity. Instead, they arise from the distinctive human capacity to stigmatize bodily differences and create unjust status hierarchies. If there is a difference from the case of racial prejudice, it is not so much that fat is preventable or remediable. It is rather that many people still openly endorse the prejudice.

---

2. We say "perhaps" because—as we mention in chapter 5—some children, especially girls, of "normal" weight also experience weight-based teasing and bullying.

The Burdens of Obesity-Related Ill-Health: Future Costs as Imperatives to Act

We make these points simply to emphasize that policies to prevent obesity cannot be justified in terms of our dislike of fat, not even in terms of a very widely shared dislike. We would also like to challenge a second and more commonly heard rationalization for obesity prevention. This consists in the future costs of treating and caring for those who will suffer from obesity-related ill-health. On this view, we should try to prevent, because otherwise we shall have to treat; lacking an effective remedy for obesity, this means treating the chronic forms of ill-health associated with it. That will prove extremely costly. There will also be economic losses when illness impairs people's ability to work.

One part of this argument is uncontroversial. It is hard to disagree with the old adage that "prevention is better than cure." Prevention is better than cure insofar as it tends to work better and spare more suffering. This is especially clear in the context of obesity because there are no safe and effective treatments, nor are any in sight (Hammer, 2010). Traditional recommendations to exercise and modify diet are notoriously ineffective, at least as weight-loss strategies; any weight lost is very easily regained. Pharmaceutical products have variable effects and unpleasant or dangerous side effects. Drastic solutions such as very low-calorie diets or gastric banding may be effective (as long as they last) but risk serious side effects. Smoking helps prevent weight gain, but its health risks are certainly greater than those of the body weight it keeps off (Flegal, 2012). In any event, because our concern in this book is with children's situation, our focus is even more strongly directed toward preventative measures.

The point at which this justification becomes problematic, we believe, is when it focuses on future economic costs threatened by obesity. Scientific and policy discussions routinely emphasize the costs that will result from people's inability to work because of ill-health, as well as the demands upon collective health-care resources. While it is reasonable to want to know how current health-care needs are arising and how expenditure has been allocated up to now, we suggest that considerable care is needed with these claims when they are projected into future decades. This is partly because such claims are bound to be highly speculative. More than this, they are morally dubious because they emphasize the wrong costs.

First, the evidence underlying projections of obesity-related costs to health services or the wider economy is weak and eminently contestable. Any such reckoning must confront many empirical uncertainties, such as those highlighted in the last chapter. It is already very difficult to estimate the proportion of current health-care expenditure that helps those with obesity-related ill-health, or the costs in economic productivity from that ill-health. Just to indicate some of the difficulties, consider how hard it would be to produce such numbers for the ill-health resulting from lack of physical activity or over-reliance on processed foods, or to meaningfully contrast these with a figure specifically relating to obesity.[3] Uncertain as such figures are in the present, they become hugely speculative when projected into the future. It is highly unrealistic, for instance, to assume that rates of overweight or obesity will increase at a constant rate, which some of the more alarming projections treat as the default scenario. Indeed, as we mentioned in chapter 1, much recent data suggest that average BMI and obesity rates have stopped increasing in many developed countries (Flegal et al., 2012; Gard, 2011a, p. 29ff; Ogden et al., 2012). Moreover, such figures tell us nothing unless they are set in context: What are the other likely increasing costs that our health and social services will have to deal with? (Compare, for example, better-founded projections of the costs involved in supporting an aging population.) What, given many improving trends in health, can we expect to save in other areas? Moreover, it is especially dubious to invoke such figures in the US context where—if money is one's concern—there is a much greater imperative to contain exorbitant health-care costs.[4]

Let us highlight another source of uncertainty in these figures, which also brings us to a moral difficulty in their use. As with smoking, which is often charged with burdening health services with the costs of treating preventable ill-health, it is not obvious which figures should enter the calculations (cf. Warner, 2000, p. 81f). What about, for example, the savings that arise from the associated early deaths—in pensions and health- and social-care needs of the old? It may sound callous to introduce those savings into the equation. The authors of one paper making "dire predictions" about the future economic costs of obesity rightly observe: "Without a doubt, health-care expenditure is high

---

3. In slightly different terms, a great deal depends on how one frames "the problem." Throughout this book, and despite our topic, we caution that obesity is *not* a straightforward problem of excess weight, but demands appreciation of many other issues that affect health and welfare. Hence our immediate point: obesity does not have straightforward costs in either human or economic terms.

4. More broadly, as Michael Gard (2011a) observes, "obesity is a very small challenge compared with the formidable and looming financial sustainability pressures that await Western health systems; pressures that are systemic in nature and have little to do with any particular disease or family of diseases" (p. 170).

for elderly people, but these costs should not be used to justify the cost-savings of dying younger, or to suggest that obesity-prevention has no benefit" (Wang et al., 2011, p. 822; see also Olshansky et al., 2005, p. 1143; van Baal et al., 2008). The reasons here are not economic, however: they are moral. To emphasize the *economic* savings from premature death is to ignore the costs borne by the individual who experiences illness and early death, and by those who care about her. But a similar callousness already lurks in alarmist warnings about the costs of obesity. Both sets of claims begrudge the costs of care and support, at the same time as they bracket the human costs of chronic illness and early death.[5] If we would prefer not to sound callous, then we should exercise restraint in lamenting projected costs in medical care or economic productivity and be unashamed to emphasize the moral case for preventing disease and suffering.

None of this is to deny that public policy is obliged to reckon with such hard and cold numbers as treatment costs, loss in working time, and the like. Certainly, present and immediate costs matter. But even they are not clearly known; and in any case, they can only be understood alongside the human costs for those who suffer the ill-health concerned. That we can expect both sorts of cost to increase unless our societies take action represents a good reason for taking preventative measures. But we should be clear both about the limits of our foresight and our principal reason for acting.[6] The primary costs associated with obesity are those borne by someone who experiences chronic ill-health or faces premature death, and those borne by his or her friends and family. And we should not forget the secondary and entirely avoidable costs of stigma and discrimination—which must be addressed not by a "battle against obesity" but by combatting stigma and discrimination.

Concern for Health and Some Complexities

As we have just indicated, the clearest and most compelling justification for obesity prevention policies is in terms of health—sometimes current health, in the case of children who are already showing signs of developing illnesses such as diabetes or other metabolic disorders; more usually, the future health

---

5. This opens the way to the barbarous claim that obesity has social costs only because societies make the mistake of offering collective healthcare provision. Thus Anomaly (2012): "some of the policies that socialize the cost of obesity and thereby make obesity reduction a public good should be changed rather than used to support further government policies that spread the costs even more" (p. 219).

6. Or as Geoffrey Rose (1992) succinctly puts it, "It is better to be healthy than ill or dead. That is the beginning and the end of the only real argument for preventive medicine" (p. 4).

of children who are currently well. Health has an excellent claim to rank as a primary good—that is, as something that everyone can agree to be desirable, no matter what else they may want to do or to happen in their lives.[7] Likewise, our concern with health reflects many other uncontroversial goods such as overall well-being, self-determination, and the capacity to actively contribute to others' well-being.

Unlike the previous two arguments for obesity prevention policies, we believe that this justification is compelling and needs little theoretical elaboration.[8] Nonetheless, there are a number of complexities associated with it that need to be borne in mind and that have implications for how we should act in support of this goal. These complexities are in addition to the empirical uncertainties considered in chapter 1, which pose questions (among other things) about how important a contribution obesity prevention can make to overall health. Here, we focus on two sources of normative complexity. On the one hand, obesity prevention is just one aspect of health promotion, and health is just one goal of public policy. On the other, obesity and ill-health may be prevented or exacerbated by all sorts of nonhealth policies or by social changes that have no obvious relation to health.

To deal with the first sort of complexity, modern societies have developed a familiar strategy—the creation of different institutions to pursue different responsibilities. Firms produce consumer goods, the different departments of government pursue different tasks, health services treat ill-health, and so on. However, this remedy comes up against its intrinsic limits when we recall the second problem: that a plethora of factors affect health. This fact poses special difficulties for policies to *promote* health and *prevent* ill-health. Recall the long-standing complaint that our health services give too high a priority to treatment as against prevention. There is a basic structural reason for this, however. Unlike treatment, health promotion and the prevention of ill-health do not fit

---

7. The term "primary good" was coined by John Rawls (1973) to describe "things that every rational man [may be] presumed to want," whatever else "he" wants and means to do with his life (p. 62).

8. As mentioned in our introduction, the more difficult theoretical question is also a political one—what are the proper responsibilities of the state with regard to public health (or more broadly, how should a society share and distribute responsibilities to judge and respond to this issue)? We will not take a strong position on those debates, and will only stress the overarching importance for public policy, that it must attempt to satisfy many different goals at once, while the proper weight to be given to those goals remains a central issue for democratic deliberation. It is also worth emphasizing that policies that appear overly intrusive or paternalistic if directed toward adults may well be unproblematic or perhaps even required when it comes to protecting children.

neatly within the purview of a single agency or institution. Hospitals, doctors, and even community health services are in a good position to react to illness. But they have very limited powers to affect those who are currently healthy or to alter factors that increase risks of future ill-health (Sacks et al., 2009, p. 84f). As all the issues identified with the term "obesogenic environment" indicate, preventative efforts must touch on many aspects of public policy.

Since health promotion and obesity prevention are not the only goals of public policy, we need to consider how well success on these dimensions combines with other goals. And we need to find ways to incorporate health within other activities of government—and indeed, of other powerful organizations, such as food companies—whether in broader integrated strategies, or more minimally as a factor that will carry some weight in each sector's policies and actions. (Compare calls for "health in all policies" or "joined-up government."[9])

Looked at abstractly, this situation poses several broad problems. These begin with the question of *priorities*. What is the relative priority of health as against other goods? What are the *costs* and *opportunity costs* of measures we might take to promote health? What opportunities do we forego in taking various measures to prevent obesity or promote health? We can try to minimize these by looking for the most cost-effective modes of action, but—since public policy needs to think in human and not only economic terms—judging costs is a difficult and contestable matter. It requires attention to the perspectives of all those who are likely to be affected (or ignored), and some sense of the priority that their claims should have. (How important, for example, are the costs to the food industry of changed labeling regulations? Or such unquantifiable costs to parents as increased anxiety about what their children are eating?) One important class of these costs can be looked at in terms of *side effects*. As we will stress below, no intervention in a complex situation can be both effective in terms of a single goal and without wider effects in terms of other goals. Almost inevitably, some of these side effects will be undesirable from the point of view of some other goal of public policy or some particular constituency.

Taking these points together, we are reminded that public policy making involves balancing many goals and making trade-offs between successes and costs on many different dimensions. Since the goal of health promotion must

---

9. As a useful (if somewhat acid) caution, compare Michael Gard's (2011b) reference to "a kind of fantasy that is actually quite common in the obesity research literature; the fantasy of a social policy context in which every arm of government is synergistically involved in the war on obesity" (p. 40).

sit alongside many goals of public policy, we need to formulate policies that are, at least, consistent with one another and, ideally, address many of those goals at once. As already suggested, this may seem to threaten only another distressing increase in complexity and uncertainty. We will argue that there is space for a more optimistic view. While it means that we are unlikely to find effective policies that prevent childhood obesity without having any other effects or side effects, it also means that we can obtain helpful guidance in formulating policies by considering their impact on many different dimensions of concern.

Multiple Goals and Single Targets

Democratic policy making has always involved overcoming many complexities. It must be made without final consensus on the goals to be achieved, and in the absence of definitive means to judge how far any particular goals are reached. One way in which democratic societies deal with these difficulties is by looking for policies that promise to contribute to many different goals at once. Inevitably this involves on-going contestation, so that policies are subject to continual revision (not necessarily refinement!). Nonetheless, the resulting compromises also enable collective action in the face of uncertainty and disagreement (Richardson, 2004; Williams, 2006).

In this section, we first consider some theoretical aspects of practical judgment—both for individuals and policy makers—and in particular its relation to multiple goals and requirements. We then turn to two examples of policies that are directed exclusively toward one goal: health-related behaviors in the first case and childhood obesity in the second. We argue that these policies face problems because of their promise to bypass the complexity of individual behavior and political decision making. To repeat, for both individuals and policy makers, this complexity arises from the need to satisfy many different goals at once. In the subsequent and final section of the chapter, we suggest these considerations point us toward a more pragmatic view of evidence and evaluation: in many cases, there can be good arguments to act, even when we are unsure that we will succeed in preventing obesity or promoting health.

Multiple Goals as the Necessary Basis for Practical Judgment

The philosopher Onora O'Neill (1998, 2004, 2007) has pointed out that multiple goals are actually vital to practical judgment—that is, to deciding how to act. If there were only one goal we wanted to achieve, then we could simply pick any effective method that lay to hand. If life were so simple, we might then find ourselves in a situation similar to Buridan's ass—our goal is just to eat hay, but we find ourselves paralyzed in doing so, because we lack criteria to decide between the different piles of hay around us. As O'Neill (2004) puts it:

> If the sole rule or principle that I sought to satisfy were that of leaving a supermarket with enough food to last the weekend I would indeed feel (and perhaps behave) like Buridan's ass—or worse. However...selecting *any* bundle of goods that would last the weekend would resolve my asinine problem. But, of course, in what we call real life I enter the supermarket not with a single aim in mind but also with many other aims and various rules, principles and laws. I not only try to get enough food to last until Monday, but also to do so quickly, without overspending, and without buying food that is unhealthy, or monotonous, disliked by those who will eat it, or produced by methods of which I disapprove....Just as equations can often be solved only when we know a sufficient number of constraints, so questions about how to act are often resolved only by taking account of a number of constraints. (p. 313f)

This is not to say that satisfying multiple requirements is always easy or even possible. Genuine dilemmas and trade-offs may occur; it may demand skill (in O'Neill's example) "to break some bad news in a way that is honest, does not undermine the confidence of the person hearing it, and yet is not so shrouded in euphemism that the message does not get across" (2007, p. 403). But although we may sometimes wish our decisions could be simpler, in general, multiple goals or requirements are both familiar and indispensable.

O'Neill's examples concern individuals. In our context, we might consider how parents need to look after the many different aspects of their children's current and future welfare, as well as taking account of their own needs and concerns. It often involves a good deal of effort and imagination to combine these many demands; some demands or desiderata will inevitably take a lower priority than others; sometimes, regrettably, parents find that it is not possible to do everything that they would like and so have to neglect some demands. From another point of view, however, the existence of many demands is also what gives shape to a person's life; without them, we would find ourselves adrift on an endless sea of possibilities, or even paralyzed like Buridan's ass. Note, too, that one of the principal lessons that children must learn as they grow up is not so much how to exercise intelligence with regard to single problems or goals, but rather how to negotiate many different requirements and spheres of life that may not be readily compatible (see further Williams, 2008).

This situation faced by individuals or parents—of multiple, possibly conflicting demands—is equally reflected at the level of public policy. As noted above, we address it, in part, by creating different departments, institutions, or agencies to fulfill different tasks—the health ministry, the competition regulator, the department of agriculture, and so on. At the same time, one of the central tasks of politics is to make sure that the activities of different parts of government and society are properly combined, without imbalances or stalemates: no task should take on undue priority; the activities of different agencies should not undermine one another.

These considerations may sound abstract, but they are of vital importance when we consider the desirability and effectiveness of different measures. Public policy properly has many ends; any policy intervenes in a complex situation where people are trying to achieve many different ends. For these reasons, direct measures targeting a single problem—"silver bullets," as it is often put—are rarely available in policy making. It is therefore politically naïve to think or act as if they might be. To illustrate, we now consider two examples of policies that have proved politically attractive because they promise to target health and obesity directly. These are information-based health-promotion campaigns and programs to measure children's weight status. While the first sort of policy clearly has an important role, we take a more skeptical view of child measurement policies. However, the point of our discussions is not primarily to assess such policies, but rather to demonstrate some problems of "single-issue" policies. In particular, there are important reasons why they are likely to be less effective than we might first hope and may have significant side effects.

Informational and Educational Health-Promotion Measures

As our first example, we would like to consider the political popularity of information-based measures in health education or social marketing. Such campaigns have been tried across many areas of public health—from smoking to safer driving to the prevention of teenage pregnancy—and continue to be deployed in most countries with a public health infrastructure. There is widespread consensus, however, that "media campaigns and promotions can have a significant impact on awareness, attitudes, knowledge, and intention to change, but generally do not change behaviors" (Swinburn & Egger, 2002,

p. 297).[10] In other words, they need to be supported by other policy measures in order to take effect.

Nonetheless, information-based campaigns still represent the most significant governmental responses to obesity in most countries. To explain this does not require cynicism about politicians' motives. One may well argue that structural interventions are liable to challenge powerful economic interests, or involve larger expenditures and longer-term commitments. Hence politicians prefer measures that focus on the responsibilities of individuals (Brescoll et al., 2008, p. 188; Food Ethics Council, 2005). Even where this has some truth, however, there are other factors at work too. The social factors affecting individual behaviors are dismayingly complex and defy simple intervention. Even where politicians are perfectly willing to take on corporate interests or act for the long term, none of the options open to them promises to have straightforward or even demonstrable effects. Educational and social marketing efforts therefore carry a ready appeal: they promise to target a specific problem, without affecting many other issues or damaging other interests.

Yet there is a quite simple reason why educational and social marketing campaigns are likely to have minimal effects. Individuals are already trying hard to satisfy many different requirements in their daily lives. (Just as conscientious policy makers are![11]) Arguably, this is especially true of parents, who must juggle many different goals and concerns against limited time and opportunities and multiple constraints. Certainly, information and advice are likely to have the very smallest effect on those persons whose opportunities are the most restricted—that is, the poorest and most disadvantaged members of our societies. Again, we do not need to reach for moralizing or cynical explanations that disparage people's willingness to act as they ought. If people are already doing the best they can given the many goals they have and the limited options they have for pursuing them, then simply telling them that—for example—more physical activity would be good for their weight or health is unlikely to change their

---

10. As Swinburn and Egger (2002) add, "An exception may be if the message is highly specific and achievable, such as a campaign targeted at changing from using high-fat to low-fat milk" (p. 297).

11. As a result, a parallel argument applies when we think about providing information to policy makers. One reason why recent calls for evidence-based policy often look more like window dressing is that policy makers must address many constituencies and priorities. This means that more information is unlikely to have much effect on their agenda or decisions, at least not unless—as sympathetic critics of evidence-based policy suggest (Head, 2008; Nutley, 2003)—it is incorporated into the demands and campaigns of different stakeholders.

behavior much. After all, the basic health messages are by now very widely known. (In this regard, one may argue that information-based health promotion has been very successful: nothing we say is meant to discredit that success!) But what is difficult to find—above all for those of lower social status and economic means—are opportunities to take enjoyable physical activity without making real sacrifices in other aspects of individual or family life. Indeed, when advice ignores these constraints it has the effect of adding insult to injury: it implies that ignorance or lack of motivation are preventing people from making the "right" choices.

In addition, it is not clear that the relative priority that information-based campaigns enjoy is without side effects. (There may also be questions about opportunity costs, which we leave open here.) As the Food Ethics Council argues in its report, *Getting Personal: Shifting Responsibilities for Dietary Health* (2005), measures that emphasize people's role in choosing healthier diets broadcast powerful claims about the proper locus of responsibilities. Instead of emphasizing the responsibilities of government to regulate agriculture and food production systems, or the responsibilities of companies in producing and marketing foods, informational campaigns imply that responsibility lies firmly in the hands of consumers (or parents, when we think about the situation of children). There is a further aspect to this, as the same report argues:

> putting the onus on individuals to choose healthy foods is counter-productive. It implies that health should be people's top priority and it underplays the other reasons why food is important. Eating and drinking play a vital part in social bonding, in distinguishing different cultures, and in shaping individual and group identities. We lose a great deal by valuing food for little but its nutrients, becoming a society of health fetishists. (p. 10)

In other words, to the extent that people accept the broader message embodied in campaigns for healthier eating, this may foster a damagingly instrumental attitude to food (diminishing the other purposes that are served by eating)[12] and an unfair division of responsibilities (something we will return

---

12. As Claude Fischler (2011) puts it, "thinking of food and eating in terms of nutrients and responsible individual choice does not seem to be helping much. If anything, the spread of obesity seems to point to the opposite, i.e., that it actually makes things worse, apparently contributing to privatizing, de-socializing and individualizing the relationship to food and eating" (p. 543).

to in chapter 3). It may be said that these are risks rather than proven costs. But since they cohere only too well with other social factors, such as widespread social anxieties around diet and health and the enormous power of the processed food industry, they demand to be taken seriously.

In any event, our main argument concerns only the relative political priority that informational and educational campaigns have enjoyed. Since parents (and people in general) have many different tasks, goals, and priorities, there are clear reasons why informational measures do not tend to alter behavior very much. As we argue in chapter 8, such campaigns have their place only within a broader set of policies that responds to all the relevant factors and priorities.

BMI Measuring or Screening Programs for Children

As a second example to illustrate the problem of "single-issue" policies, consider programs to weigh and measure all children in a given state or country. On the face of it, these look like measures that directly target childhood obesity, without affecting other domains of life and policy. Several states in the United States have legislated to require schools to measure the BMI of all pupils and to report this information to parents (Levi et al., 2012, §3). Similarly, the United Kingdom has set up the National Child Measurement Program (Dinsdale et al., 2012; NHS Information Centre, 2012). Nonetheless, these policies have proved controversial—doubtful in their effectiveness and cost-effectiveness, dubious as regards their side effects and opportunity costs. The reasons for this are easy to make out and could well have been foreseen. (For further critique in the UK context, see Evans & Colls, 2011; in the US context, see Cogan et al., 2007; in the Canandian context, see MacLean et al., 2010.)

Such policies typically have a double rationale: surveillance and screening. On the one hand, they survey the extent and distribution of childhood obesity, and whether this is increasing over time. On the other, they represent direct interventions in children's and families' lives: report cards or measurements are given to parents, which should alert them that their child is overweight or obese, and may be combined with advice as to how to respond to this fact.[13] Such a double justification may seem to fit well with our broader argument that public policy must try to achieve different goals at once. This will be true, however, only to the extent that (a) both goals are necessary and

---

13. Some might be inclined to put "fact" in scare quotes: recalling our discussion in chapter 1, this is a fact that only *appears* simple.

(b) likely to be achieved by this means; and that (c) the policy does not have undesirable side effects or significant opportunity costs. Unfortunately, there is good reason to doubt that any of these basic conditions is met.

Let us begin with the first rationale, concerning comprehensive information about childhood obesity. Universal knowledge of children's weight and height suffers the double problem of being "too much and not enough." First, it is *too much* information; we do not need to know every child's BMI, nor exactly how this varies from year to year, to judge the extent and distribution of childhood obesity. This requires only systematic sampling. A universal measurement policy is simply disproportionate to the goal of judging the extent of childhood obesity: it is effective but not cost-effective. But that is just one side of the problem. The second aspect is that universal BMI measurement does not provide *enough* information: height and weight are very simple and selective measures. Any scientifically responsible study of childhood obesity will examine many, many more factors—children's diet, parenting style, social class, physical activity patterns, health-related biomarkers, such as measurements that bear on metabolic syndrome, and so forth.[14] Simple BMI measures become merely simplistic if they are taken to supply knowledge about health and well-being. In short, such a policy generates far too much of one type of information, and much too little of other crucial forms of information.

It might also be said that parents are unlikely to be unaware of their child's weight, both absolutely and relative to other children. This point is often countered by evidence that parents of overweight or obese children tend to downplay their child's weight, for instance, by adopting various common euphemisms ("solid," "well-built," "puppy fat," and so on)—and indeed by evidence that measuring programs may lead to greater accuracy in parents' assessments (West et al., 2008). Nonetheless, it is important to recognize that parents have an obvious and immediate responsibility as regards their child's self-image—to avoid stigmatizing labels and not to encourage a child's self-consciousness about, or dislike of, his or her body.[15] It might be borne in mind, for example, that it is not so much fatter children, as children who feel self-conscious about being fat, who tend to be the targets of weight-related bullying or social isolation (Brixval et al., 2012; Fox & Farrow, 2009). April

---

14. Here, again, we would like to acknowledge our debt to the IDEFICS study consortium (www.idefics.eu; Ahrens et al., 2011a), which has involved exactly this sort of study of thousands of European children.

15. Parents' sense of this is conveyed well by the interviews reported in Backett-Milburn et al. (2006).

Herndon (2010) nicely expresses the bind parents face as a result of an emphasis on body weight: in the "current political climate…acceptance of a large child seems risky…despite the fact that such unconditional love and acceptance seems to be what is most needed and wanted by children" (p. 346; see also Schwartz & Puhl, 2003, and the case discussed by Ludwig, 2012).

As this suggests, it is not clear that parents really need accurate information about their child's weight status. First, such an emphasis conveys a message that weight is an important index of health and that weight loss is desirable in itself—so that inappropriate and perhaps counterproductive dieting and weight loss measures may be encouraged. Neumark-Sztainer et al. (2008) found that "parents who recognized that their children were overweight were more likely to encourage them to diet. Parental encouragement to diet predicted poorer adolescent weight outcomes 5 years later, particularly for girls" (p. e1495). Second, weight-related measures are not adequate indices of whether a child is at risk of developing health problems or should change his or her behavior to improve his or her health. As just indicated, one needs to look at a wide range of factors such as developmental trajectory, various biomarkers, and so forth. All of these may be problematic in a thin child, just as they may not be in a fat child. The problem is only that they cannot be assessed by a simple report card on height and weight. Again, the information being given to parents is "too much and not enough." *Too much*: there is no reason why parents need to know their child's BMI or place on a developmental or percentile curve. *Not enough*: weight-related measures are only meaningful alongside many other items of health-related information, as interpreted by medically trained personnel. (See also Barlow & Expert Committee, 2007; Cogan et al., 2009; MacLean et al., 2010.)

Perhaps more important still, note that there is not much use in highlighting some children as special targets for concern unless corresponding interventions are available (Westwood et al., 2007). Measuring programs, and indeed other measures that emphasize body weight, risk placing a significant burden on parents. Unaccompanied by suitable guidance, the responsibilities implied remain indeterminate and hence may foster anxiety or prove counterproductive in various ways. Alternatively, advice and interventions may seem rigid or unrealistic or interfering. To avoid these and other dangers, child measurement must be integrated with genuinely accessible and supportive measures for the family. Here it matters greatly what sort of wider health infrastructure is available, as well as what degree of control parents have over their environment and that of their child. Many families are affected by poverty, poor housing, unsafe environments, parental ill-health, or other forms of social disadvantage—in such cases, change will be that much more difficult to make. Worse, demands for change from health or social services may carry a coercive edge: that is, parents may hear—even where this is not intended—demands for change as accompanied by the threat of "or else (your child will be taken from you)."[16] Even where this is not the case, the general fact is that desirable changes are still likely to run counter to many aspects of children's and parents' lives in modern societies—the "obesogenic environment" that we discuss further in chapter 6.

Looked at in this light, child measuring programs no longer appear simple or straightforward, nor are they cheap or risk-free. In the context of generous and well-thought-out support for parents and children, they may seem to have a rationale. But in this case there will be no need for them, since there will already be many ways to identify children who are showing poor health or indicators of future health problems. Where support services are more meager, there is much to be gained from enhancing those services—and little from child measurement policies. Obesity is not the direct target that such policies take it to be.

Responding to Empirical and Normative Uncertainty at Once

Our decisions about what to do are generally structured by many different goals and constraints. So policies that aim to achieve just one goal may be defeated by the fact that people are themselves trying to balance many different responsibilities, as well as the variety of factors underlying health and illness. At the same time, there may be—and invariably are—reasonable disagreements about the relative priority that various goals should have, and who should take responsibility for them. Modern Western societies give individual adults a great deal of freedom to decide these matters in their individual lives. One might feel that they are rather more judgmental of the balances that parents strike.[17] When it comes to public policy, however, every society needs to

---

16. Compare Annette Lareau's findings on the strikingly different perceptions of working- and middle-class parents in this regard (2011, p. 231). For another face of state coercion in a context of inadequate support, see also Bridgeman (1998). Aptly titled, "Criminalizing the one who really cared," this discusses the tragic death of Christina Corrigan and the prosecution of her mother for child neglect.

17. Thus Frank Furedi's book, *Paranoid Parenting* (2002), which highlights the battery of institutional expectations and (supposedly) expert advice to which parents are subjected, leaving many feeling anxious, judged, and disempowered.

arrive at *collective* judgments—compromises that settle relative priorities and combine many different goals.

In this final section, we take up the problems of empirical uncertainty raised in chapter 1 alongside the problems of normative uncertainty discussed in this chapter. In practice, these uncertainties tend to appear side-by-side and may leave us feeling that we face an impenetrable thicket of unresolved questions and insoluble problems. We would like to develop a more optimistic view by suggesting that the appropriate strategy is to focus on policy measures that promise gains on many different dimensions. If we do so, we may also take a more pragmatic view about the evidence supporting a policy on any particular dimension—not least, whether it will reduce children's obesity rates. This is not to say that we should not try to obtain robust evidence, let alone disregard it when it does come to hand. But we will need to take account of evidence on many different dimensions and from many different sources, and accept that it will rarely have the certainty or precision that experts naturally hope for.

One way of highlighting the issues here is to observe the double problem attending recent calls for "evidence-based" policy making. Inevitably, this phrase has a somewhat rhetorical ring. While no one disputes that policies must take account of the empirical evidence, or indeed that social ills should be ameliorated, there are so many relevant sources of knowledge and so many possible ways of assessing priorities that the supposed parallel with "evidence-based medicine" breaks down immediately. As Adam La Caze and Mark Colyvan (2006) argue, the goal of medicine is relatively easy to specify, whereas the goals of policy are multiple and contested. Likewise, there is "depth and stability [in] our understanding of the causal process or mechanism [for pharmaceutical interventions]," and we have "the capacity to meaningfully isolate the intervention of interest when testing drugs" (p. 6).[18] Neither is true in the policy domain. Instead, the challenge is to maintain and adjust a plethora of policies (institutions, regulations, initiatives) and to consider whether to develop and introduce another policy (institution, regulation, initiative). Together, the empirical and normative issues—empirical uncertainty and multiple sources of evidence, normative disagreement and the plurality of individual and social goals—simply defeat any parallel with

---

18. It is perhaps worth adding that matters are also less simple when we consider overweight and obesity, even at the level of individuals. Insofar as they are not pathologies, they do not represent clear targets in their own right; nor are they preventable or treatable by a single intervention.

medical treatment. As we hinted in chapter 1, even when our concern is with population health, it makes no sense to view policies as if they were remedies administered to the body politic.

In the first place, policy making must draw on many different types of evidence, at many different stages, among many actors who have quite different powers, perspectives, and priorities. Consider, for example, a perennial difficulty of the policy process concerning knowledge of the effects of different policy measures. Policies are implemented—often imperfectly and unreliably—in a constantly changing environment. They are rarely single measures and often involve a whole suite of interventions. Each policy always operates alongside many other policies. All of them are undermined or supplemented in their effects by an enormous number of factors that lie beyond policy makers' control or even purview. Calculating their costs, even the direct financial costs of implementing or maintaining a policy, is never easy. The opportunity costs—all the things that had to be foregone in order to implement the present policy— are never really calculable. Likewise, gauging the effects and side effects of a policy is possible only in quite limited ways, never mind comparing them with the (side) effects that alternative policies might have had. To obtain any sort of handle on how a policy measure is affecting a given issue, and what sort of other effects it may be having, requires careful attention to many different voices and types of evidence.[19] We might reasonably hope that experts can provide us with at least some points of certainty. But just as often they show us how many questions are still open and why certainties are so hard to come by. Politically, the need is for public debate and the inclusion of many voices in the policy process so that the real complexities can become clear to all parties (Lobstein, 2005).

However, it is not just a question of disagreement, limited perspectives, or even ignorance about a complex set of facts. Second, policy making must also consider different views as to what goals are desirable, their relative priorities, and which responsibilities should be borne by whom. For these reasons, we have stressed—however disconcerting this may seem in a book about childhood obesity—that neither obesity prevention nor health promotion are the sole goals of public policy. If obesity prevention were an end in itself or—still more implausibly—the overriding goal of public policy, then we could select

---

19. Or as Harry Rutter (2012) puts it, "There is a fundamental epistemological difference between the rigorous EBM [evidence based medicine] methods that can differentiate between two treatments, and the kinds of research that are able to identify effective, sustainable approaches within complex adaptive systems" (p. 657).

and assess policies by how they affect obesity rates.[20] There would still be practical difficulties, given the empirical uncertainties and the difficulty of judging what would have happened in the absence of a given intervention. But at least we would have a clear problem and a clear index of success. However, in the policy domain, as elsewhere, there are often very good reasons to forego action *in spite* of evidence for its effectiveness. The outlawing of processed foods would certainly reduce average BMI levels; a little more realistically, an abrupt end to agricultural subsidies might well have some effect in the same direction (at least in the United States; see Wallinga, 2010). These are not options because they would be far too disruptive of other goods we value. In other words, we can neither choose nor evaluate policies with only one end in view. Nor, for the same reason, is there ever just one policy "in question." Governments, like individuals, are always pursuing many different courses of action at once; different groups and organizations depend on these in ways that are difficult to oversee.

Both empirical and normative issues set significant limits on the role that particular sorts of evidence and particular forms of expertise can play. Evidence is always partial: it needs to be incorporated into a larger picture. It also requires judgments about how important and desirable are the different effects, costs, and risks to which that evidence testifies. Similar issues apply to expertise. This is naturally selective: a person can be an expert only on particular issues. Likewise, expertise has a natural tendency to prioritize particular problems and goals. As a result, it should be no surprise—nor even a cause for disappointment—that political decisions are often at odds with expert evidence and prescriptions. This is not to deny that such oppositions may reflect problems in the policy process: ignorance or ideology on the part of policy makers, misplaced hopes of a "quick fix," or the power of vested interests, for example. But as we have underlined in these opening chapters, there is also a very good reason why evidence and expertise should not dictate policy. Evidence, in the strict sense that experts naturally hope to provide and draw on, has an important place—but *not* pride of place. This is partly because emerging evidence about complex phenomena—whether we take a multifactorial condition such as obesity, or any

---

20. This would clearly be incredible. But observe that cost-effectiveness analyses implicitly consider policy choices in terms of just two goals—to achieve certain effects and to minimize (or contain) expenditure. The many other goals of policy are left hidden in the wings, waiting on whatever resources are not devoted to the issue at hand. (See also Richardson, 2000, and note 21.)

intervention in a large society—is rarely decisive. It is also because expert evidence cannot supply a comprehensive perspective: even expert collaborations, such as those involved in public reports about how to respond to obesity, focus mainly on one matter of concern. As such, expertise must bow to what are ultimately political questions—above all, we suggest, those concerning priorities and the allocation of responsibilities that we stressed in the book's introduction.

However, there is one upshot of this situation that should, we believe, be welcome to those who wish to address a social problem, whether or not they are experts in a particular aspect. If certainty about achieving a desired effect is not enough to dictate policy—and it never is, so long as there are other goals that we also need to consider and weigh—then lack of certainty cannot dictate policy either. So we should not be deterred from intervening by, for example, the reasonable disagreements discussed in chapter 1 concerning which interventions will succeed in preventing childhood obesity. For example, there are good reasons to think that increasing children's walking and cycling to school will make some contribution to preventing childhood obesity. But this is not certain. Nor is it certain that particular policy measures can bring about higher rates of walking and cycling. We may not even be able, after the fact, to demonstrate that policies definitely worked on either dimension. But a case for action can still be made where we can point to other likely benefits—such as reduced car use or opportunities for children to develop greater independence—and if we can find a way to integrate policy proposals within existing divisions of responsibility—such as local authorities' duties to foster safe built environments.[21] In other words, so long as we have a reasonable basis for believing that a proposed policy will have desirable effects in some of these dimensions, and not have damaging effects in others, then we do not need unambiguous evidence—either prospectively, to show that it will "work," or retrospectively, to demonstrate that it did. This does not mean ignoring new evidence as it becomes available. But it does remind us how, and how often, we manage to act successfully in the face of uncertainty about the facts and disagreement about our aims.

---

21. Compare the example of "walking school buses" as discussed by Carter et al. (2009). On their analysis, this turns out not to be a cost-effective childhood obesity prevention measure. But as the authors also note, "some interventions have multiple objectives that include broader traffic congestion, community and environment goals.... When a share of costs is attributed to these broader objectives, then cost performance is improved" (p. 419). There may still be better ways to intervene, but assessing this is a matter of broader political judgment.

Concluding Remarks: "Something Must Be Done"—But *What*?

In this chapter, we have highlighted what we consider to be the main *normative* problem facing the choice and assessment of policies in the context of obesity prevention. Obesity prevention is just one aspect of health promotion; health is just one of the proper goals of public policy. Political decision making needs to take account of all of these goals, in the context of enormous social complexity and demands from many different constituencies. Particular agencies, such as health services, are unlikely to be in a position to make effective interventions on their own.

One response to this complexity is to look for policies that target health behaviors or childhood obesity directly, even if only to a limited degree, because everyone can agree that "Something Must Be Done." We have considered two examples of policies that promise to do this. Looked at more carefully, neither delivers. The complex range of factors that affect people's health and children's development mean that apparently direct interventions are unlikely to have significant effects and may have undesirable ramifications. Nonetheless, such policies have obvious political appeal, for voters no less than politicians. So it often seems that for every new accident, threat, or misfortune, we hear calls for another law or policy—"Something Must Be Done," "There Ought to Be a Law Against It," and so on.

The basic problem with this mode of response arises from a striking similarity in the situation that faces both individuals and policy makers. Individuals, parents, health professionals, and public officials must all grapple with many different priorities and uncertainties; rarely is it reasonable to give one task absolute priority or to assume that all the facts are in. Failure to recognize this complexity can generate problems on all sides. Voters or media voices may show impatience and make unrealistic demands for direct solutions. Entrepreneurial experts may hawk pet solutions around the media. Health professionals and agencies, while aware that many factors frame individual choices and behaviors, may nonetheless feel—again, understandably but not always realistically—that advising individuals about how to live more healthily (or even informing parents of their child's BMI) should suffice to bring about the desired outcome. At any rate, they may find that such channels are all that are open to them in the absence of social and political will to act more broadly. Politicians, in turn, face structural incentives to take measures—and above all, to be *seen* to take measures—that clearly target a matter of public concern. While it may require political courage to challenge vested interests or to take measures with no short-term pay-offs, it also involves courage to resist simplistic demands of the "Something Must Be Done" variety.

Those demands need to be resisted because public policy must take account of many different goals—obesity prevention and public health, social equity and economic prosperity, and a host of other things besides. Some of these may be agreed priorities for many parties. Others may seem more or less important depending on, for example, different parties' existing responsibilities or interpretations of complex evidence. The proper response, we have suggested, is to try to balance as many different goals and address as many different problems as possible, without demanding certainty that we will succeed on each count. In slightly different terms: when we face a wicked problem, there is no question of solving it with a single policy. What *is* possible is a thoughtful exercise in what one might call "coalition building": of creating and adjusting policies so that we address a range of different issues. This does not mean trying "to solve all the problems of society."[22] But it does mean accepting that there are many problems, none of which permits a single "solution" but all of which we have the power—and responsibility—to address.

---

22. Hawkes (2008, p. 1204), as quoted at the start of this chapter.

3 CHILDHOOD OBESITY AND PARENTAL RESPONSIBILITY

The language of personal responsibility plays a prominent role in public discussions of obesity, as it does in discussions of diet and other health-related behaviors (Food Ethics Council, 2005; Kim & Willis, 2007). This is reflected in public opinion research, which has noted a pervasive attribution of individual responsibility for overweight and obesity (Fuemmeler et al., 2007; Hardus et al., 2003; Okonkwo & While, 2010; Potestio et al., 2008). The words "responsible" and "responsibility" are often related to simple and sometimes simplistic lines of thought that emphasize individual choice and suggest that duties, risks, and costs ought to be borne by individuals—not least by those persons who are already overweight or obese. It is questionable how far adults have the abilities and opportunities to minimize risks of becoming obese, or to successfully lose weight if they are. In any event, such claims have little purchase when we consider the incidence and prevention of childhood obesity. Clearly, younger children themselves lack the abilities and opportunities to control their diets and lifestyles. Instead, public and policy discussions naturally turn to the responsibilities of parents, which form the topic of this chapter.[1]

Despite the simple uses to which it is sometimes put, the concept of responsibility is complex. For this reason, we begin with two short sections that aim to clarify two key aspects. The first concerns two important meanings of responsibility. The second concerns how responsibility connects with judgments about the benefits and burdens that people should bear. The following sections then consider three substantive questions about parental responsibility. First, we examine the complex relation between causation and responsibility. We will argue that actors who play a causal role in an outcome such as childhood obesity are not necessarily morally

---

1. There is an important question about the opportunities and responsibilities of older children or adolescents. As discussed in the introduction, we will say relatively little about this, and we set it aside in this chapter entirely.

responsible. Often they are—but this is not always the case. Instead, what matters is whether an actor has a duty to prevent such an outcome, as well as a reasonable opportunity to do so. We then raise some questions that arise when one judges that some parents really are at fault for their child's overweight or obesity. Without denying that there are such cases, we suggest that the practical implications of this point are relatively limited. In the final section, we consider the wider question of who should bear responsibilities to address childhood obesity. While there are no simple answers, we argue that it is important to remember that who takes responsibility for what is also a question about social cooperation. We illustrate this point by considering the responsibilities of food and drink companies as they relate to parents' responsibilities.

Although we will take issue with some ways in which "responsibility" and "parental responsibility" figure in discussions about childhood obesity, there are two starting points that we believe all contributors to this debate can share. First, no one doubts the importance of parental responsibility. It is a child's parents—or in particular circumstances, other adults who have taken on this role—who must bear primary responsibility for overseeing a child's upbringing and welfare. While there are tragic cases where this does not happen, it is also clear that most parents take this responsibility extremely seriously. Second, no one believes that parents should bear this responsibility alone. Bringing up children is always a matter of social cooperation. In many respects, this cooperation is a marked success of Western societies—schools, health organizations, commercial bodies, and the state all share in the duties owed to children.

Nonetheless, this consensus leaves room for disagreement about the exact scope of different responsibilities; there are occasions when one actor may be felt to interfere in another's sphere of responsibility or to neglect their own; and there may be dispute as to who, if anyone, should assist if one party lacks the resources or opportunities to fulfill his or her responsibilities. All these problems matter when we think about childhood obesity. Many changes in Western societies over the past decades have had the effect of depriving parents of support, or undermining their efforts, in ways that encourage childhood obesity. Sometimes advice—or blame—from those concerned with obesity may be perceived as interference, or may fail to take account of a person's (or an institution's) wider situation. Other actors, as we suggest in the final section, may not be in a position to support parents, even if they would like to. Our broader argument in this chapter, then, is that when we think about parental responsibility, one of our leading concerns must be the social arrangements that enable responsible parents to succeed in their task, and other actors to support their efforts.

Retrospective and Prospective Responsibility

The words "responsible" and "responsibility" have several meanings, but two aspects are central. The *Oxford Dictionary of English* (2010) defines responsible as:

1. Having an obligation to do something, or having control or care for someone, as part of one's job or role...
2. Being the cause of something and so to be blamed or credited for it.[2]

That is, responsibility is either *prospective*, in referring to on-going and future obligations or duties, or *retrospective*, in referring to past actions to which liability or credit may be attached (Williams, 2012b). So we may ask who is responsible for the rise in childhood obesity, in the sense of asking who is to blame: this is to take a retrospective, or backward-looking, view of responsibility. Equally, we may ask who is responsible for preventing or addressing childhood obesity: this is to take a prospective view, concerning current and future responsibilities.

We will discuss below how prospective and retrospective responsibilities are connected, and their relation to causal factors. But let us note one simple and intuitive connection at the start. In attributing prospective responsibility, we usually imply that retrospective responsibilities may follow from this. For example, a person may have a duty to look after a certain item. Should this item get broken then a duty to repair or replace or compensate would usually arise. That is, if a person fails in her prospective responsibility to take care, this will give rise to a retrospective responsibility. We will argue that this connection is key to understanding responsibility: it is people's prospective responsibilities that provide the basis for attributions of retrospective responsibility. At the same time, it is crucial that people—and collective actors such as companies and even the state—are accorded the resources and powers to fulfill their prospective responsibilities.

---

2. It also notes a third meaning: "(of a job or position) involving important duties, independent decision-making, or control over others...capable of being trusted" (see Williams, 2008). We will also have this sense in mind when we speak of "responsible parents."

Responsibilities as Benefits or Burdens?

It is natural to think of responsibilities in terms of burdens and penalties, for two reasons. First, when we consider backward-looking responsibilities, our thoughts generally turn to various burdens—liability to blame and feelings of guilt or remorse, duties to compensate, and various sanctions including punishment. Second, when we consider forward-looking responsibilities, our attention is naturally drawn to the requirements that these involve—constraints upon our actions that limit our freedom and require us to expend time and energy and resources in particular ways.

Such a negative view is mistaken. With regard to the first point, it is important to remember that when we act well or rightly, we are often owed various benefits from others—the payment or wage for a job well done, praise or gratitude for having done our duty or gone beyond its call, and so on. More broadly, when others recognize us as having acted rightly, we experience the wider benefit of participating in social life and enjoying good relations with them. That others may respond in ways we dislike to our failures to act well, or that we ourselves may feel guilt or remorse for failing to act well—these negative possibilities are just the counterpart to opportunities to interact with others on good terms.

The same point also applies to the sense of constraint implied by prospective responsibilities, especially when they are framed in terms of "duty" or "obligation." For example, no one would deny that parental responsibilities are extremely demanding. But as a social relationship—as opposed to a matter of mere biological causation—parenthood just *is* taking care of one's child. Most parents bear the costs involved without even thinking of them as such, because the parent-child relation is such a unique privilege and valued opportunity. A parallel point can also be made about the responsibilities of companies. Especially in the US context, companies and their lobbyists tend to present regulatory requirements as burdens or impositions. This one-sided view, as we suggest below, obscures the role that requirements can play in enabling corporations to act responsibly by parents and children.

When we are asking, then, how responsibilities should be distributed, or how to allocate responsibilities for addressing the increasing incidence of childhood obesity, it is important to remember that this is not primarily a matter of sharing an onerous task or, still more negatively, deciding who has failed and should now pay the price for this. That is just a small part of a much wider question regarding the opportunities, rewards, and cooperation that are possible when responsibilities are fairly distributed and actually fulfilled. Of course, this understanding may not make it easier to decide immediate practical questions as to who should do what. But it sets those questions in a wider context, and may help us to approach them in a more hopeful and positive spirit.

Individual and Parental Responsibility for Childhood Obesity

Having made these introductory points, we divide the remainder of this chapter into three sections. In this section, we consider the role that causation plays in generating responsibilities. We argue that the primary question is never really causation, but rather what different actors' prospective responsibilities are. In other words, although it may be tempting to think about responsibility in terms of individuals—who caused what?—this approach cannot succeed. Instead, we must consider the distribution of prospective responsibilities among different actors. Our discussion here may seem, to some readers, too ready to excuse parents whose children become obese. Second, then, we consider the practical implications of judgments that some parents *are* to blame—and argue that these are unlikely to be straightforward. Finally, we turn to prospective responsibilities. As we have noted, there is universal agreement that parents should bear primary responsibility for their child's welfare and upbringing. Deciding the scope of this responsibility and who else should contribute are more difficult. We will—throughout this book—not attempt to offer definitive answers. But by considering a concrete example of the tension between parents' duties and the actions of food and drink companies, we hope to illuminate the issues at stake.

A common approach to responsibility is to look at it retrospectively, in terms of who brought about what outcome. It is often true that those who cause a negative outcome should be encouraged to change their behavior, or be blamed or penalized. So it is natural to think that if someone is causing a harmful effect, then she should also be considered responsible for it. Thus we might seek to attribute responsibility for childhood obesity in line with the causes of childhood obesity, so far as we have reasonable knowledge of these. Of course, this is not just about apportioning fault and blame. It is usually thought of as a way to identify those who should bear responsibility for addressing childhood obesity by altering their behavior to avoid or reduce its incidence. In more abstract language: we would be looking for causes in order to attribute retrospective responsibility, and deriving prospective responsibilities from these.

Insofar as it focuses on what an individual does or brings about, this line of thought is attractive by virtue of its apparent simplicity. But as we have been at pains to stress, simplicity is not available here. The causal pathways involve endless chains and complex interrelations—recall, once more, the famous "spaghetti diagram" from the UK Foresight report on obesity (reproduced in the opening pages of chapter 1). So our judgment goes awry if we latch on to just one or a few causes. However obvious a particular factor seems to us, it will only be part of the story, and perhaps not the most important part.

There is also a more disreputable reason why the causal story may seem tempting. As Schwartz and Brownell (2007, p. 84f) note, members of Western societies tend, when other people fail in some way, to attribute blame to them. Yet when a person herself fails, she may well blame this on her circumstances. Conversely, we tend to explain others' successes in terms of their external circumstances—while preferring to see our successes as due to our own efforts and qualities. Social psychologists have consistently demonstrated this systematic bias and call it the "fundamental attribution error"—we wrongly attribute others' failures to their own faults, just as we wrongly attribute our successes to our own virtues.[3] Such beliefs about causation—that it is due to individuals' over-eating and lack of exercise or to parental failings—often rationalize moral condemnations of obese people or the parents of obese children.

Underlying this is the broader problem that causes are themselves always caused, and many causes are not human actions. Even if one person clearly caused an outcome, we can still ask what caused him to act as he did. When epidemiologists identify various factors that make our societies "obesogenic," they are following Geoffrey Rose's (1992) well-known precept to consider "the causes of causes" (ch. 7). It may be parents who purchase food for the household and feed their child, and who therefore play a role in causing their child's obesity, but their actions are hardly unaffected by further causes. Food purchasing is constrained by income; employment opportunities and other factors affect the time available to shop, prepare, and share meals; and, as we stress below, market forces and state interventions determine food availability and prices. As we observe in chapter 4, systematic inequalities in the

---

3. The phenomenon is discussed in all textbooks of social psychology, for example, Aronson et al. (2012). For detailed discussion in the context of obesity, see Crandall and Reser (2005).

distribution of overweight and obesity suggest that these causal factors impact more heavily on poorer people and families.

The difficulties involved here can also be brought out by looking at the frequent mismatches that occur between causation and responsibility. An actor may be responsible for certain effects that she did not cause; equally, she might not be responsible for them, even where her actions did play a causal role. Both facts point to serious issues with regard to childhood obesity and the responsibilities of parents and other actors.

Start with the case where a person or organization plays no causal role. There are often cases where we ascribe responsibility to actors who are *not* causing an outcome: we may blame or punish someone for *failing* to intervene. For example, it might be argued that in some countries, statutory bodies are failing to protect children from obesity. In such cases, the problem is not that statutory bodies are playing a causal role in the increase in childhood obesity, since the problem is precisely their lack of action. Instead, they are judged to be failing because they have a duty—in our terms, a prospective responsibility—to uphold children's welfare. In other words, it is not causation that identifies who should be held responsible, or who should take steps to address the problem. Instead, who is (retrospectively) responsible depends on a morally more fundamental question: who had a duty to act in the first place?

Looking at the matter from the other direction, it is equally true that a person's causal role need not generate claims of moral responsibility. We do not necessarily expect someone to take account of *all* the effects of his actions—however likely or foreseeable those effects, and however many opportunities there were to act differently. For example, in setting up a business that is a rival to someone else's, I may well foresee that my competitor will go out of business. But unless I have engaged in illegal or sharp practices, I would not normally be deemed responsible for his losses. My responsibility is to run a competitive business, not to worry about my competitor's prospects.[4] Such judgments turn on substantive moral claims about who should do what and who should bear what risks (Ripstein, 1999). Similar arguments are often offered in the context of childhood obesity and need to be evaluated on a case-by-case basis. For example, food manufacturers can hardly deny that they play a causal role in the over-consumption of energy-dense foods, since they

---

4. We discuss below the importance of regulatory measures that may impose additional responsibilities on companies. For the moment, the point is just that business responsibilities cannot extend to taking account of competitors' prospects—that would abolish competition itself.

supply these goods in the first place. As we consider below, however, they may argue that these foods are safe in moderation, and that individual consumers and parents are responsible for failing to balance their diets.[5]

In the case of parental responsibility, the first point (about omissions) may sometimes apply, but the second (concerning consequences that are not one's responsibility) will not. Parental responsibility is peculiarly demanding partly because parents cannot ignore anything that affects their child's well-being, development, and future prospects. For this reason they may, as in the previous example of state agencies, sometimes be reproached for failure to intervene, even if they do not actively cause their child's weight gain. Nevertheless, we obviously do not expect parents, or other actors, to do the impossible. For example, where someone lacks a reasonable opportunity to act differently, this mitigates the (prospective) claim that he has a duty to act in a particular way and the (retrospective) claim that he was responsible for adverse effects resulting from his action. Consider, for example, a mother's decision to breastfeed, which some studies have shown to reduce the risk of overweight and obesity (e.g., Hunsberger et al., 2012). Robertson et al. (2007) point out that

> whether a woman breastfeeds her child, or not, can be influenced by a combination of factors including: her economic situation; access to paid maternity leave; her access to optimal maternal services and health care; her level of education; aggressive marketing by baby food companies; her cultural environment; and her personal beliefs. (p. 60)

Many factors may lead a mother *not* to breastfeed, then, even if she believes that breastfeeding would be preferable for her child's health. Those same factors may well affect our judgment of what it is reasonable to expect of her— that is, they may suggest that she does not have a responsibility to breastfeed, all things considered.[6]

We can put this point in terms of the multiple goals and requirements that we discussed in chapter 2. To blame the mother for failing to breastfeed

---

5. Such an argument is evidently risky from a public relations perspective. More common, companies prefer to focus on the importance of physical activity and exploit—or even foster— continued uncertainty about the relative roles of diet and physical activity in causing obesity.

6. We cite—and contest—this example partly because responsibility for a child's obesity is so often attributed to the mother, understood as the primary carer who feeds her children (Herndon, 2010). Maternal blame is an all-too-common theme in media reports of childhood obesity (Maher et al., 2010).

would be to assume that she should treat the possible benefit to her child's health as more important than everything else she needs to take account of, such as her own interests or those of other family members (Holm, 2008). But like anyone else, she cannot treat a single claim as if it had absolute priority. This highlights another reason why the fundamental attribution error comes so easily. We are all, from our individual perspectives, familiar with the constraints and goals that we must take account of in our daily lives. But it is easy to look at other people's lives in the abstract, without appreciating all the different factors they must reckon with. When we have a particular priority in mind—such as preventing childhood obesity—it is very easy to attribute failure to parents whose children become obese. On a more careful reckoning, however, we may well find that parents are doing the best they can to address many different priorities at once.

We will stress below that circumstances may make it very hard to balance and combine different priorities. Consider, for example, a problem that many parents of already overweight or obese children must grapple with. As we mentioned in chapter 2, in discussing child measuring programs, most parents are—quite rightly we think—anxious not to imply that their child should be self-conscious about, let alone ashamed of, his or her body. Medical (or other) professionals—whose responsibilities are focused more narrowly upon physical health—may feel that these parents should clearly recognize the child's overweight or obesity and address it as a priority. The problem for parents is that the two concerns pull in opposite directions. As Schwartz and Puhl (2003) write,

> the implicit message in encouraging [dietary] restriction may be internalized by the child as saying that there is something wrong with his or her body. In a society that stigmatizes obesity, how can parents encourage healthful eating without generating feelings of shame in the child and self-blame for the obesity? (p. 64, see also p. 67)

Depending on the particular personalities of parents and child, and the circumstances in which they find themselves, it may be impossible to address both issues satisfactorily. In this case, stigma and prejudice against fat persons have put responsible parents in a position where they cannot act responsibly. It has become impossible for them to adequately address all the factors affecting their child's development.

Looked at more theoretically, these considerations show that claims about retrospective responsibility cannot be based simply on what a person causes. Instead, they hinge on claims about what we may expect of somebody, morally speaking. Looked at more practically, the point is not only that attributions of blame may be unfair or out of order. More importantly, they reveal a crucial question concerning the distribution of responsibilities. If children are not faring as well as they ought, while parents are doing the best they can, who should take responsibility for remedying the situation?

Aren't Parents Sometimes Genuinely to Blame?

We have emphasized the problems of aligning causation and responsibility. Despite playing a causal role, a person may not be responsible for the negative effects of her actions; mitigating circumstances may imply a duty to assist rather than to reproach. Some readers may feel that we have been one-sided in offering arguments that mitigate parents' responsibilities. We do not mean to deny that people are sometimes genuinely to blame for their actions and choices. Some parents surely do feed their children badly, for example, despite having the wherewithal to feed them well. Nonetheless, we do think it is worth considering what is gained by emphasizing this. After all, the point is not merely to apportion blame, but also to prevent childhood obesity and promote children's health (alongside, as we have already stressed, many other goals). With this in mind, we want to make three points, beginning with the most alarming cases of alleged failure.

We will say very little in this book about one of the most publicized issues around childhood obesity. This concerns legal decisions to remove extremely obese children from their parents. Such cases naturally grab media attention and arouse controversy, but they are also rare and extreme. To remove a child from his or her parents is a desperate measure, made still more so by the chronic underfunding of children's social services in most Western countries. Relevant here will be our degree of certainty that the parents are truly harming their child to a greater degree than removal and statutory child care would, or indeed whether the parents are doing anything wrong at all (see Campos [2004, ch. 7] for the sad and cautionary example of Anamarie Regino in New Mexico, taken from her parents by social services simply on the basis of dramatic weight gain). Also relevant will be the child's wishes where he or she is able to express a view. (See Bridgeman [1998] for a tragic teenage case, albeit not framed in terms of removing the child.) Apart from emphasizing the extremity of using state coercion and taking a child from his or her home, the main point to note is that these are primarily cases of child protection. This represents a highly complex area in its own right, with no simple choices or easy options. The child's weight is simply an occasioning factor—and most likely not the only one—that needs to be dealt with in a child protection framework. As such, these cases lie beyond our scope here.[7]

Less drastically, an emphasis on some parents' failings may be taken to imply that someone should actively decide which parents are to blame and single them out for reproach and sanctions, or require them to alter their behavior. Taken in the abstract, this is clearly not likely to be helpful or effective. Rebukes are unlikely to be well-taken, while requirements would be hard to specify and enforce. In line with our emphasis on the distribution of responsibilities to act, we need to ask a more practical question: whose responsibility might it be to blame parents and set them straight? As soon as this question is posed, it is obvious that such interventions could only be fair or effective where someone already has a clear relation to, and responsibility toward, a particular family. Lacking these, there could never be adequate knowledge of the family's situation and any reproaches would be presumptuous and interfering. Where there is such a relationship—for example, where professionals have been working with a family—it may, on occasion, be appropriate to reproach parents or even to threaten sanctions if they fail to alter their behavior. But these are complex questions of judgment. In particular, they require attention to the many other goals and responsibilities that parents have, how well they are attending to these, and the particular difficulties they may be facing. In other words, such judgments only make sense within relationships or institutional frameworks whose basic orientation is to support parents, not to oversee or blame them.

More modestly again, an emphasis on parental failings might correspond to frequent media or public health messages suggesting that some (many?) parents aren't doing enough. (Although they sometimes overlap in practice, note that this is a different message than giving parents advice on healthy lifestyles. One may inform without hectoring—just as one may hector without informing.) Arguably this sort of response has been quite common over the last decade or so. After all, talk is cheap: commentators gain the appearance

---

7. For balanced discussion focused on obesity see Varness et al. (2009) and Viner et al. (2010); Murtagh and Ludwig (2011) offer a more judgmental view. On broader questions of the state's role in child protection see Archard (2003, esp. part III: The State).

of care and concern for free—and well-intentioned parents pay the price in terms of anxiety and guilt. As for the few parents who are not, for whatever reason, genuinely trying to do their best by their children—they are hardly likely to heed such reproaches. In other words, this sort of response is neither effective nor fair. However culpable a few parents may be, most problems arise by virtue of the economic, social, and environmental changes that have affected children and families over the past decades. It is these changes that deserve our sustained attention.

Sharing Responsibility to Address Childhood Obesity

We now turn to the allocation of responsibility to parents, and more generally, the extent to which responsibilities to care for children should be shared with other actors. In particular, we explore some consequences of situating parents' responsibilities within a wider context, illustrating this with the example of companies that market food and drinks to children. As we emphasized at the start of this chapter, there is universal agreement on two principles concerning responsibility for children: First, it is parents—or on occasion, guardians who have stepped into this role—who bear primary responsibility for a child's upbringing and welfare. Second, this responsibility is nonetheless shared with many other actors, such as schools, health professionals, and state agencies. Conflicts are certainly possible here—for example, parents may experience some well-intentioned interventions or bureaucratic measures as interfering or misplaced. In general, however, the second principle does not contradict the first. To do their job well, parents depend on schools, voluntary organizations such as religious or social groups, the services of many companies, and a wider framework of safety and security provided by civic cooperation and a legal framework.

There are large moral and philosophical questions about the exact scope and bases of these responsibilities, which we can only gesture at here. For example, some authors underline the fact that parental responsibility is peculiarly stringent: as well as requiring continued attention to every aspect of a child's development, there is also, as Anne Alstott (2004) puts it, "no exit," at least not until a child has grown up. In all fairness, then, this is a role that demands support from wider society. This contention is supported by an argument offered by many other authors: parents perform one of the most fundamental human duties by securing the continuity of our societies (Archard, 2004; Engster, 2010) or, more abstractly, allowing us hope for the future.[8] Bluntly put: if we fail in raising the next generation, then all our other achievements must be in vain.

Of course, some voices baulk at the characterization of raising children as a shared task. Responding to Hillary Clinton's (1996) invocation of the phrase, "It takes a village to raise a child," Bob Dole (1996) once claimed, "it does not take a village to raise a child. It takes a family to raise a child."[9] Since few of us now live in villages, there is literal truth here. But that was hardly Dole's point, and his words represent mere point-scoring because they evade the basic issues. If families are not achieving everything that we might hope of them—so that many children are becoming obese, or suffering forms of preventable ill-health—then we are left with a stark choice. *Either* we write off many parents as simply not up to the task—with all that implies for their children's future health and prospects—*or else* we admit that parents require assistance. So we must look for changes to existing social arrangements that will be both fair and effective in enabling children's healthy development.[10]

Obviously, this still leaves an enormous amount open. What should count as a fair and effective division of responsibilities? What priority should we give to children and their future prospects as against (for example) the rights and interests of adults in the present? Nonetheless, such a perspective overcomes the limitations of discussions that focus on the responsibilities of only one set of actors, such as individual parents. If other persons or organizations, or the ways we structure our social life, are undermining a cooperative venture (such as the upholding of children's health) it is unfair and even hypocritical to focus on individual parents and expect them to "step up" (Holm, 2007, 2008). Only when all actors do their part within a given cooperative scheme is fairness upheld. In this case, both benefits and burdens are reasonably shared, and a shared task can be performed effectively. Nonetheless, we need to bear in mind that similar considerations apply to other actors, such as food and beverage companies. There will, for example, be little merit in blaming commercial forces, if other factors prevent companies from playing a more constructive role.

---

8. For a literary perspective on this point, see P. D. James's (1992) novel, *Children of Men*, also memorably filmed by Alfonso Cuarón (2006).

9. British readers might also recall Margaret Thatcher's (1987) pronouncement: "There is no such thing as society. There are individual men and women, and there are families."

10. As we argued in the previous section, an apparent "middle way"—where our "assistance" takes the form of reproach and hectoring—has little to recommend it.

To explore some of the issues here, we would like to consider an argument made by Schwartz and Puhl (2003). They suggest that successful cooperation has not yet been established with regard to children's nutrition and make a provocative contrast with questions of safety in marketing products to children. Legal provisions uphold strict safety standards with regard to the sorts of toys that manufacturers sell to particular age groups. Similarly, manufacturers recognize that it is in their interest to be seen to behave responsibly. This creates, as Schwartz and Puhl put it, "an environment where parents, the legal system and product manufacturers are working toward the same goal of protecting children" (p. 57). As a result, simply by following straightforward guidelines as to whether toys are appropriate for their child's age, parents can trust that they will not risk their children's health. By contrast, Schwartz and Puhl suggest that there is an absence of such cooperation in the case of processing and marketing food. This creates "the challenge of parenting in a toxic food environment" (p. 58).[11]

So far as food manufacturers are concerned, however, there are several respects in which the parallel does not hold up. On the one hand, any processed food must already meet quite stringent standards with regard to purity, permitted additives, labeling, and so on. Manufacturers may therefore argue that they are already fulfilling their responsibilities in terms of the safety of particular food products, just as toy manufacturers do. On the other hand, they may argue that so far as problems do exist in children's diets, these do not arise from particular food products. Instead, these problems result from overall patterns of consumption, and ultimately from consumer choices: that is, they result from failings on the part of parents and others who cater for children. Food processing, manufacturing, and marketing clearly play a causal part in children's diets; but the moral responsibility—so the argument goes— lies with parents and consumers.

Despite these differences from the case of toy safety, we believe that Schwartz and Puhl's argument still deserves to be taken seriously and exemplifies our wider points in this chapter. Their argument concerns the overall food environment, as opposed to individual food products. While this may not be "toxic," it clearly represents—as we discuss further in chapter 8—a situation where the most readily available and widely promoted options pose risks to children's

---

11. Or as David Ludwig (2007) puts it, "Why should [parents'] efforts to protect their children from life-threatening illness be undermined by massive marketing campaigns from the manufacturers of junk food? Why are their children subjected to the temptation of such food in the school cafeteria and vending machines?" (p. 2327).

health. No individual product need be unsafe, but the combined effect is to undermine parents' attempts to ensure their children have a healthy diet.

However, there is no simple line from this conclusion to a judgment that food companies are to blame. As we emphasized in the last chapter, different actors have many different responsibilities to fulfill, just as parents need to look after the many different aspects of their child's welfare (as well as their own!). On the face of it, companies are in a position to do many things that might reduce or prevent (childhood) obesity. They might, for example, desist from targeting children with hyper-palatable foods, deep-fried confections of low-grade animal products, and large servings of sugary drinks. But the same mitigating argument that applies to many parents also applies to companies: if a course of action is impossible, or blocks other essential goals, then it would be unfair to demand that an organization undertake it.

At the start of this chapter, we pointed out that the concept of responsibility is commonly associated with constraints and burdens—but that it also relates to opportunities, powers, and rewards. This double-sidedness often shows up in debates concerning regulation for food labeling or food composition, such as bans on trans-fats. Critics present such measures as limitations on freedom—as limits on companies' prerogatives or consumers' liberties. Advocates point out that such restrictions create new freedoms, such as consumers' ability to know more about products or freedom from worry about artificial and unhealthy ingredients. Critics, in turn, point to additional costs to consumers or suggest that consumers' gains come at the price of legitimate commercial freedoms.

This familiar back-and-forth often misses an important point, however. We suggest that well-designed regulation is enabling for *companies*, as well as consumers and parents. Although cynicism comes easily here, there is no doubt that many who play key roles in food and beverage companies would prefer not to undermine children's health and well-being. But the poor record of voluntary initiatives and "self-regulation" amply demonstrates that companies are not in a position to prioritize this concern.[12] Clearly no company can survive—which is to say, remain profitable and avoid take-over—unless it takes seriously the fierce pressures on price from retailers and similar pressures in terms of short-term profits from stock markets.[13] These pressures also

---

12. We discuss the limits of self-regulation further in chapter 8, in terms of children and advertising.

13. Both sets of pressures, in turn, reflect the way companies and stock markets are structured and regulated—again, these problems are especially acute in the US context (Mitchell [2001]; see also Roberts [2008] on specific pressures within the food industry).

make companies highly sensitive to the cost implications of regulatory measures (exacerbating the natural tendency we have mentioned, to think about responsibilities in terms of burdens and constraints). To these points should be added a further consideration. Companies are not in a position to admit their *inability* to cooperate with parents to support children's health, as the contortions of their public relations activities so often testify.[14] Ironically, this also creates incentives to resist regulation, since—looked at in a certain way—regulation conveys a powerful condemnation: companies cannot be trusted to act well of their accord.

In other words, companies are caught in a triple bind: unable to support children's health as many of their executives and employees might wish, unable to admit this, and hence unable to welcome measures that would assist them to act more responsibly. Commercial pressures continue to dictate the promotion of hyper-palatable, over-processed, and energy-dense foods and drinks to parents and children. In presenting themselves as responsible actors that care about children's health and welfare, companies find themselves committed to incompatible tasks. Against this background, appropriate regulatory measures can enable companies to act more responsibly, since they remove the competitive advantage gained by business practices that undermine parents' attempts to uphold their children's health. While it is hardly a simple panacea, we believe that it helps to look at regulation from this rather different angle: not as a restriction or even a penalty imposed on actors who have failed to show voluntary restraint and social responsibility, but instead as an enabling measure that recognizes the impossibility of fulfilling incompatible goals.

Obviously, these points are highly schematic and leave open many questions about the fairness and effectiveness of different regulatory possibilities—not to mention their relative priority and how they may complement or conflict with other desirable goals, or the responsibilities of other actors, such as schools or local government. But we hope our discussion may still illustrate three complementary points. First, an absence of constraints may allow some actors to impose additional responsibilities and burdens upon others, while the imposition of constraints may enable those same actors to act more responsibly. Second, to act responsibly depends on an effective scheme of social cooperation. In the case of companies, we do not want them to cooperate as such: in the marketplace, the paradigm instance of cooperation is a

---

14. See Stones (2012) for a memorable example of these.

cartel. Instead, the challenge is to make sure that competition does not lead them to act in ways that undermine parents and damage children's health. A fairer balance is surely possible, but it requires a wise regulatory framework. Finally, since responsibility depends upon cooperation, to focus on the responsibility of just one set of actors is usually unfair. Much as some may wish to blame them, food and beverage companies can reasonably plead—though they are unlikely to say this in public—that commercial responsibilities cause them to undermine parents and prevent them from marketing responsibly to children. And although some voices seem keen to blame parents—especially those whose children are already overweight or obese—we need to remember how often those parents are doing their level best to negotiate an environment that is, if not "toxic," at least riskier than need be.

Conclusion

There is no doubt that parents bear important responsibilities with regard to childhood obesity, as part of their broader duty to care for their child's welfare. Doubtless, too, there are ways in which parents sometimes fail to do all that they can or should. But parents must take care of many other aspects of their child's upbringing; and both they and their children live within a complex causal web that has generated an increasing incidence of childhood obesity. To focus on parental responsibility, with much popular and policy discourse, is to disguise this complexity. Brownell et al. (2010), argue that "an overemphasis on personal responsibility and mislabeling actions that enhance personal choice as 'government intrusion' prevents or stalls needed policy changes that can help people be responsible" (p. 383f). We have argued that this point applies particularly when we think of actions designed to enable parents to fulfill their responsibilities. And we have also suggested that it applies to commercial actors: well-designed regulation can enable companies to act more responsibly—even when they publicly reject the need for such interventions. Both parental and commercial responsibility depend on a societal division of responsibilities, and we should be loath to attribute blame without examining whether this cooperation is properly established.

Of course, it is not just changes in food and drink markets that have affected parents' situation over the past decades. For example, higher levels of road traffic, together with higher expectations about safety, mean that parents often do not let children play outside without direct supervision. Likewise, in a society of strangers, parents often feel that they cannot rely on other adults to look out for their children—thus the sociologist Frank Furedi (2002) discusses a "breakdown in adult solidarity" vis-à-vis children (p. 11f). In this situation, parents find that if their child is to be both safe and active, they have to do much more to make this possible. Again, one may feel that the cumulative result now represents an unfair burden on parents—it has become more difficult for them to combine the different aspects of bringing up a child, together with other important aspects of life such as work and relaxation. In other words, responsible parents have been put in a situation where it has become more difficult to act responsibly. To redefine the responsibilities of other actors, such as companies, educational bodies, and government, and to ensure that they are not caught between incompatible demands, remains a central task for citizens and policy makers alike.

4 CHILDHOOD OBESITY INTERVENTIONS, EQUITY, AND SOCIAL JUSTICE

While equality is an important consideration in many areas of social policy, we often think it is particularly important in the realm of health: even in societies that are quite tolerant of inequalities in income and wealth, there is a presumption that health inequalities are problematic (Daniels, 2008). In countries across the world, various indicators of health—such as life expectancy, morbidity, and mortality rates—exist across a social gradient, with disadvantaged groups suffering worse health outcomes than those in better-off groups (Stuckler & Siegel, 2011). Childhood obesity is no exception. In many industrialized countries, childhood obesity is more prevalent among children from low socioeconomic status (SES) families and in many ethnic minorities. This may further exacerbate other health inequalities and also inequalities in other areas, such as unemployment—not least because of weight-based discrimination.

In this chapter, our central question is how considerations about equality and inequality should affect the policies to tackle childhood obesity. Interventions that can successfully reduce childhood obesity among disadvantaged groups could also make an important contribution to the reduction of social inequalities in health, if disadvantaged groups benefit to a greater extent from these interventions than their more advantaged counterparts. However, with respect to many public health interventions—such as health promotion messages—researchers have been concerned that low SES groups do not benefit to the same degree as higher SES groups. We conclude by considering how concerns about inequality should be reflected in the design and evaluation of childhood obesity interventions. Before entering into these discussions, however, we begin by summarizing some current evidence on differences in the prevalence of childhood obesity in different groups.

Inequality and Childhood Obesity

In many countries of the developed world, overweight and obesity—including overweight and obesity among children—are more common among the disadvantaged, such as low-income groups or ethnic minorities (Department of Health Public Health Research Consortium et al., 2007; Kuipers, 2010). In a comparison of 35 high- and middle-income countries, Due et al. (2009) found that in most countries there was a social gradient in the prevalence of obesity among adolescents, although absolute prevalence among children differed across countries. Studies use a variety of different indicators of SES, which may account for some of the differences in results across different studies (Johnson et al., 2011). When dealing with children, a further problem is that many traditional indicators of SES are not directly applicable and, instead, SES is measured with reference to family, community, and/or school characteristics (Johnson et al., 2011). These difficulties notwithstanding, childhood obesity has been linked to poverty (Phipps et al., 2006), deprivation (Kinra et al., 2000), and lower levels of parental education (Lamerz et al., 2005).

In addition to inequalities in the incidence of childhood obesity, obesity may also have a greater impact on quality of life on those in lower SES groups. Kinge and Morris (2010) found that the negative impact of obesity on health-related quality of life measures was greater in adults from lower SES groups. They also found that the negative effects of overweight and obesity on health-related quality of life were greater for women than for men (see also Muennig et al., 2006). This reflects the well-known tendency for different sorts of disadvantage to cluster and even reinforce one another. While, to our knowledge, this has not been studied with respect to children, these results suggest that data on social differences in the prevalence of obesity may understate further inequalities in the impact obesity has on individuals' quality of life.

There are also suggestions that inequalities in childhood obesity are still increasing, even where overall trends appear to have leveled off (Gard, 2011a, ch. 3). For example, in the United Kingdom, inequalities in childhood obesity have grown more pronounced, since the incidence of obesity has increased most among children from poorer backgrounds (Stamatakis et al., 2005). Similarly, data from a study of adolescents in California concluded that socioeconomic inequalities in obesity were increasing, with this increase occurring more consistently among adolescent boys than girls (Babey et al., 2010). The authors suggest that this may be the result of anti-obesity efforts failing to reach adolescents in low-income families, echoing the familiar concern that at least some types of public health interventions fail to reach disadvantaged groups, thus exacerbating inequalities—an issue we discuss in more detail below.

Inequalities in overweight and obesity rates have also been found for children in some ethnic minority groups (e.g., Saxena et al., 2004). Other disadvantaged groups may also be disproportionately affected. For example, some studies find higher obesity rates among migrant children relative to nonmigrant children of similar social status.[1] Family structure may also matter. While this has not been examined extensively, it appears that children in single-parent families have higher rates of obesity than children in two-parent families (Gibson et al., 2007). Finally, gender remains an important consideration with respect to childhood obesity as well, as social inequalities have been found to be more pronounced in girls than boys (Kinra et al., 2000).

What do we know about the reasons for these inequalities? Just as with questions that surround the etiology of (childhood) obesity, there is no consensus as to why, exactly, childhood obesity rates in developed countries tend to be higher among lower socioeconomic groups. Studies have explored a range of factors that might be implicated in producing such inequalities.

Many commentators argue that environmental factors play a substantial role in creating social inequalities in obesity rates among children. Given that important resources such as healthy foods and safe environments for physical activity tend to be much more accessible for more affluent groups, it is not implausible that these factors contribute to inequalities in obesity rates. Johnson et al. argue that because obesity rates decrease as the socioeconomic environment improves, it is not poverty as such but, rather, risk factors that are distributed incrementally across the socioeconomic spectrum that explain social inequalities in childhood obesity (Johnson et al., 2011). For example, because children from low-income families appear to watch more television, they may not only be more sedentary but they may also be exposed to more advertising for foods than children in higher income families (Kumanyika & Grier, 2006). We discuss the role of obesogenic environments in more detail in chapter 6.

A number of studies also consider differences in the choices made by parents in different socioeconomic groups. For example, one study suggests that medium and high SES parents tend to have three fixed meal times, that

---

1. See Kirchengast and Schober (2006) for data from an Austrian study and Will et al. (2005) for a German study. A review of European studies is provided by Labree et al. (2011).

they require their children to taste all foods provided, and that they are more restrictive when it comes to their children's consumption of sweets. Low SES parents, on the other hand, seem to be less restrictive when it comes to unhealthy foods, and they may also see food as a means of demonstrating to their child that they are not disadvantaged (Haerens et al., 2009). Also, differences in breastfeeding practices may contribute to social inequalities in childhood obesity, as breastfeeding has been argued to be protective against overweight in children (Woo et al., 2008). Parents' choices, of course, as we emphasized in chapter 3, are influenced and constrained by environmental factors. For example, income inequalities may explain why, relative to low SES parents, food purchases of medium and high SES parents are more influenced by quality than by price, and that these parents seek out healthier foods that rely less on cheaper commodity foodstuffs (e.g., Haerens et al., 2009). (We take up this issue again in chapter 7, where we consider the role of food prices in childhood obesity and the use of taxation and/or subsidies as a policy response.)

Similarly, parents' attitudes and beliefs have been considered as a possible cause for the unequal incidence of childhood obesity. Johnson et al. (2011) note that, relative to lower SES individuals, higher SES adults tend to be more health conscious, have a greater belief in individual control over weight and health, and see lifestyle as more important in determining health outcomes. Of course, such beliefs may be justified or reinforced by the greater opportunities for choice that tend to exist for those on higher incomes, in professional careers, or with higher education levels.

Another possible reason for social inequalities in the incidence of childhood obesity is that low-income mothers or mothers with low levels of education perceive their children's weight differently than mothers in more educated, higher income groups, often failing to recognize their children as overweight or obese. (It is mothers, rather than parents, who are the focus of these studies: e.g., Baughcum et al. [2000]; some studies, however, do not find such a link: e.g., Carnell et al. [2005].) While these differential perceptions are often viewed as a problem, it is crucial to bear in mind that family discourse about weight concerns is problematic and can have negative consequences for children. For example, one study finds that even parental comments about weight and eating that were meant to encourage daughters to maintain a healthy diet and weight were linked to higher body image dissatisfaction and disordered eating (Kluck, 2010). In a different study, girls who reported that their parents encouraged them to be physically active so as to facilitate weight loss were found to be more concerned about their weight and to have higher BMIs than girls who had not been encouraged to lose weight in this way; neither did this kind of encouragement lead to higher levels of moderate to vigorous physical activity (Davison & Deane, 2010). Thus, even well-intentioned advice that parents give their children to protect them from obesity can have harmful and counterproductive consequences.

Further, low-income parents appear to have a greater tendency to resist growth charts that health professionals present in order to indicate that a child is overweight (Hughes et al., 2010), and they may use other indicators to determine whether or not they should be concerned about their children's weight. For example, qualitative studies suggest that they tend not to worry as long as children are physically active but become concerned if children's activity decreases, or when their self-esteem suffers because of weight-based teasing from their peers (Hughes et al., 2010; Jain et al., 2001). In the literature, this is again often seen as a problem that needs to be addressed (e.g., Baughcum et al., 2000). However, given concerns about the validity of weight categories for children (as discussed in chapter 1), as well as the problems associated with focusing on weight loss rather than healthier behaviors, it is not clear how, or indeed *whether*, parents should react to their children's "official" weight status. Relying on criteria more obviously and directly linked to their children's well-being may not, after all, be such a bad strategy.

Finally, it is important to remember that, as with other questions around childhood obesity, our knowledge about which kinds of interventions can actually reduce disparities in the incidence of childhood obesity is limited. However, as we emphasized in previous chapters, it does not follow that we should not attempt to reduce such inequalities. The case remains for measures that seem promising and that we have good reason to expect to be beneficial in other regards, especially if we can monitor their effects and ensure that their overall effect is positive.

Justice and Health: What Are Health Inequalities, and When Are They Unjust?

How exactly should the existence of these inequalities be assessed? And what grounds the view that these inequalities constitute an injustice? In this section, we briefly situate questions around inequalities in childhood obesity in the broader context of debates about health inequalities. We highlight some of the complexities in deciding what makes particular health inequalities unjust and indicate how these apply to the childhood obesity context.

Health inequalities, and possible strategies for their reduction, have received increasing attention at both international and national levels. At the global level, the WHO's report on the social determinants on health (Commission on the Social Determinants of Health, 2008; Marmot et al., 2008) has attracted considerable attention. The European Union has stated its concern about health inequalities both within member states and between them (Commission of the European Communities, 2009; Ministry of Health and Social Policy of Spain, 2010; see also Mladovsky et al., 2009), and a number of national governments have also drawn attention to health inequalities in their countries (e.g., see Department of Health, 2008, for a UK perspective).

However, despite the apparent consensus that health inequalities are problematic and that their reduction should be an important goal for governments and other public bodies, there are debates about how health inequality should be conceptualized and when, or to what extent, health inequalities are actually problematic. In this section, we explore the distinction between just and unjust health inequalities and discuss several criteria that have been emphasized, with particular reference to the context of childhood obesity.

In the health literature, it has become commonplace to use the term "health inequality" to capture *all* health inequalities, whereas "health inequity" denotes those health inequalities that are unjust. As Kawachi et al. (2002) describe the terminology, "health inequality is the generic term used to designate differences, variations, and disparities in the health achievements of individuals and groups...health inequality is a descriptive term that need not imply moral judgment." Health inequity, on the other hand, "refers to those inequalities in health that are deemed to be unfair or stemming from some form of injustice" (p. 647).

Perhaps one of the most influential accounts of how the line between health inequality and health inequity should be fleshed out comes from Margaret Whitehead (1991, 1990). Central to her account is that, to be unjust, health inequalities must have been *avoidable*. Thus, health inequalities resulting from "natural, biological variation" (Whitehead, 1991, p. 219) would not be considered inequitable. This suggestion has been influential in policy contexts. For example, the recent Report by the Commission on the Social Determinants of Health states that "where systematic differences in health are judged to be avoidable by reasonable action globally and within society they are, quite simply, unjust. It is this that we label health inequity" (Commission on the Social Determinants of Health, 2008, p. 26; see also World Health Organization, 2010, 2007). By contrast, to the extent that the lower average life expectancy of men compared to women reflects biological variation, it would not—on Whitehead's account—be seen as unjust.

A related proposal to distinguish fair and unfair health inequalities consists in the extent to which such inequalities are *amenable to intervention*. Norheim and Asada argue that "the relevant distinction is whether the institutions of society can respond adequately to a disease or not" (Centers for Disease Control and Prevention, 1999). Thus, whether or not a particular inequality is unfair will also depend on the availability of treatments or policies that can help address the health condition in question. A similar judgment appears to be implicit in Daniels's (2008) account, when he notes that "to the extent that [the] social determinants [of health] are socially controllable, we clearly face questions of distributive justice" (p. 81).

On some accounts, health inequalities are unjust if they have *unjust causes*. For example, Daniels's (2008) influential account of justice in health distinguishes fair from unfair inequalities according to whether or not they were caused by an unjust distribution of the social determinants of health. This has also been defended by political philosophers as a more general criterion in deciding whether particular inequalities are unjust (e.g., Young, 2001). The basic premise at work here is that if inequalities are socially caused, then there is a more urgent case for institutions or individuals to address—or rather, redress—the resulting inequalities (Pogge, 2002). By contrast, on other accounts of distributive justice, the distinction between inequalities that result from social rather than natural causes is irrelevant and does not affect the urgency attached to remedying the inequality (e.g., Segall, 2009).

Finally, some theorists suggest that inequalities are not unjust if they can be linked to the exercise of *individual responsibility*. On such an approach, health inequalities resulting from "lifestyle choices," such as smoking or sports accidents, would not be unfair. As we discussed in chapter 3, individual responsibility for health represents a complex and controversial issue. At any rate, in the present context, we are concerned with children, who generally are not regarded as responsible for the choices they make because they are not (yet) autonomous (Archard, 2004; Scarre, 1980). Even if it can be argued that health inequalities resulting from adults' choices are not unfair, the same cannot be said about children.

These brief remarks illustrate some of the difficulties around the identification of unfair health inequalities. For the purposes of this chapter, we do not need to take a position on this larger debate. The unequal health outcomes resulting from an unequal prevalence of childhood obesity across groups are likely to count as unjust on all the criteria that have been can-vassed to distinguish unjust health inequalities. The fact that childhood obesity has only recently emerged as a public health concern suggests that it is an avoidable outcome and should be, at least to some extent, amenable to intervention. The evidence reviewed in the previous section indicates that the prevalence of obesity is greatest among children from disadvan-taged groups, suggesting that it is linked to inequalities in other spheres. Finally, as mentioned above, children generally cannot be held responsible for the choices they make with respect to food and physical activity. There are therefore very good grounds for regarding inequalities in childhood obesity as notably unjust. So there is a special need for policies that can successfully tackle rising obesity rates among disadvantaged groups, par-ticularly low-income and ethnic minority groups.

It is also worth recalling one reason why health inequalities, including inequalities in the incidence of obesity and overweight, are taken to be espe-cially problematic. They may exacerbate existing health inequalities as well as leading to, or exacerbating, inequalities in other spheres. Anand notes that "health is regarded to be critical because it directly affects a person's well-being and is a prerequisite for her functioning as an agent. Inequalities in health are thus closely tied to inequalities in the most basic freedoms and opportunities that people can enjoy" (Anand, 2002, p. 485). Such a concern is particularly pronounced in relation to effects on education and labor market outcomes. In addition, since obesity is a highly visible and stigmatizing condition, further inequalities can be expected to arise in all social spheres. For example, Puhl and Heuer (2009) review the available evidence of discrimination against the obese in employment, health care, and housing. We examine questions of stigma and discrimination in more detail in chapter 5.

It also worth emphasizing why children and their health are of particular importance when we are concerned with the reduction of social inequalities in health. First, large socioeconomic inequalities as well as health inequali-ties have been identified among children (Mielck et al., 2002). Second, child-hood represents a "key life stage," as exposure to disadvantage at an early age can have "lasting effects on socioeconomic status and on health in adult life" (Mielck et al., 2002, p. 144). Importantly, even when particular health condi-tions are not yet apparent among children from lower SES groups, exposure to certain socioeconomic conditions in childhood can increase the likeli-hood of such conditions in adulthood. For example, it has been suggested that even when obesity rates among children are not greater among lower SES groups, as adults they are more likely to experience obesity (Power et al., 2003). Thus, commentators argue that childhood is a "particularly critical period for interventions designed to reduce health inequalities" (Mielck et al., 2002, p. 147).[2]

Reducing Social Inequalities in Childhood Obesity: Assessing the Impact of Interventions

Friel et al. (2007) propose a policy agenda that views obesity through an "equity lens." This requires that prevention strategies take account of the fact that

> obesity—and its unequal distribution—is the consequence of a complex system that is shaped by how society organizes its affairs. Action must tackle the inequities in this system, aiming to ensure an equitable distribution of ample and nutritious global and national food supplies; built environments that lend themselves to easy access and uptake of healthier options by all; and living and working conditions that produce more equal material and psychosocial resources between and within social groups. This will require action at global, national, and local levels. (p. 1242)

While we very much agree with the view expressed here, in this section we would like to draw attention to some complexities and trade-offs that arise when policies or interventions try to address inequalities.

We need to consider, first, the possibility that health promotion activities can increase social inequalities in health. Experience with public health initiatives in other contexts, such as smoking, suggests that affluent groups often benefit more from health interventions than worse-off groups;[3] this has also been noted as a possible problem for obesity interventions (Swinburn, 2009). In one study, the effects of a family-based intervention were found to be less for children from lower SES relative to higher SES families (Langnäse et al., 2004). An Irish school-based intervention program seemed to have a smaller effect on schools in deprived areas relative to more affluent areas (Friel

---

2. As noted in our introduction, we do not think this justifies the lack of priority sometimes attached to inequality as it affects adults. Our point is only that there remain reasons to be especially concerned with children's situation.

3. See Saelens et al. (2012) for a review of evidence regarding such effects and Sallis and Glanz (2006) on such effects in the context of nutrition interventions.

et al., 1999). When this is the case, interventions may exacerbate, rather than reduce, social inequalities in health.

Evaluations of these kinds of interventions should, therefore, include an explicit assessment of its impact on (in)equality. In particular, we must first identify those groups who are likely to benefit less from the intervention or to suffer disproportionately from its negative effects. In the context of childhood obesity interventions, this is likely to include lower SES families and marginalized or vulnerable groups, such as single-parent families or migrants (Ahrens et al., 2007). We may also want to consider effects on female versus male participants as well as on individuals with particular health problems. Note, further, that some measures may benefit children who are not overweight but disadvantage those who are. Greater emphasis on physical activity in schools, for example, may be good for many children; many obese children, however, may not feel that they can participate in such activities without shame or fear of ridicule.

One way to respond to this problem is to remain with broader or "universalist" approaches that aim to improve the health status of *all* children but also try to address the barriers that prevent disadvantaged groups from benefiting (Mielck et al., 2002). For example, to deal with financial barriers faced by low-income families, interventions may have to provide parents not only with suggestions about how to prepare healthy meals but also with advice about how to do so on limited budgets. Likewise, suggestions that children join sports clubs or play in gardens or nearby parks may not be affordable for or applicable to lower-income families. Instead, campaigns could pay particular attention to how physical activity can be maintained where access to playgrounds or green spaces is limited. Since poverty is often experienced as a source of shame in itself, such strategies demand careful thought, and remind us how important it is to involve disadvantaged groups in planning interventions and implementing policies. Similar concerns apply in the context of ethnic minority groups, who may be reached more easily when interventions are adapted to take account of particular cultural beliefs or traditions. Indeed, linguistic or cultural barriers may mean that supposedly universal provision fails to reach some groups. Advice on healthy eating that presupposes a particular cuisine, for example, is likely to seem irrelevant or exclusionary to ethnic groups with different eating habits. Again, in order to overcome such obstacles, there is clearly a need to work with the communities concerned to ensure relevant messages are conveyed through accessible channels.

Another strategy to respond to the concern that interventions may inadvertently increase social inequalities in health is to target interventions at particular groups. For example, interventions may focus on children in lower socioeconomic groups, or from particular ethnic backgrounds, or even on those children who are already overweight or obese. While such targeted strategies may well be appropriate and attractive when we are seeking to eliminate inequalities in health outcomes, one of the general dangers they face is that they may stigmatize or at least "mark out" a particular group.

Consider the proposal, recently made in the United States, that food stamps for those on low incomes should no longer allow for purchases of sugar-sweetened beverages (see Shenkin & Jacobson, 2010, for discussion). Commentators have cautioned that such restrictions contribute to the stigmatization of those on low incomes. The executive director of the New York City Coalition Against Hunger, for example, suggested that the proposal "was based on the false assumption that poor people were somehow ignorant or culturally deficient" (McGeehan, 2011; see also Barnhill, 2011, for further discussion). It is difficult to assess the extent to which interventions do indeed have these implications but any such effects are clearly problematic. Still, it may be the case that concerns about stigmatizing effects are outweighed by the health improvements involved—for example, if they do in fact reduce soda consumption among those reliant on food stamps. Nonetheless, we suggest that given the overall message conveyed by such a policy—that the government should decide what poor people may consume while leaving wealthier persons to make their own decisions—it should bear a heavier burden of proof. That is, there would need to be convincing evidence—going beyond the relatively weak likelihoods often provided by epidemiological data—that it will result in clear health benefits.

The possibility that targeted interventions may help improve health but can also exacerbate stigmatization highlights the more general concern that improvements in individuals' health are sometimes brought about in ways that impose burdens on them in other domains. As we explain in more detail below, this makes it particularly important that we attempt to capture as far as possible the full effects of particular interventions, going beyond a narrow focus on weight-based measures or even measures that focus on health more broadly.

A further trade-off that policy makers must consider when devising strategies to reduce social inequalities in health is that interventions may bring about improvements for one disadvantaged group by imposing burdens or harms on a different disadvantaged group. In the present context, we have to be particularly concerned about interventions that impose burdens on *parents* in disadvantaged groups so as to bring about benefits for their *children*. Given the importance of early childhood for health outcomes later in life as well as social mobility, policies that shape the choices parents make on behalf of their children could be highly effective. Nonetheless, such interventions might interfere with parents' choices in ways that impose significant costs or limitations on them. We address this concern in more detail in chapter 6.

Finally, at a more general level, the promotion of health equality may come into conflict with other important goals. Policy initiatives to reduce social inequalities in health generally have opportunity costs, as the resources used for such policies could instead be spent on the pursuit of other objectives. In other words, as we noted in chapter 2, both individuals and policy makers need to balance many different goals against one another—health does not enjoy absolute priority over other goods. Weighing the priority of health and health equality against other important goals is, of course, a highly complex task. It means considering values that are very different in nature and that may be judged more or less important by different people and groups.

How should judgments about such trade-offs be made? Some authors have tried to combine these (and other) considerations into a single index to help us balance different values and to facilitate policy decisions. For example, Norheim (2009) argues for an approach that makes explicit our judgments about how equity and efficiency concerns should be traded off against each other. However, there remains no clear or widely accepted way to judge trade-offs between competing aims such as those of reducing social group inequalities and improving average health (Daniels, 2008). When faced with the difficulty of finding the "right" balance between competing objectives, philosophers often propose a greater role for involving the public in such decisions, through consultation and deliberation procedures that go beyond more political, democratic channels (see, e.g., Daniels & Sabin, 2008).

What do these concerns and the difficulties in balancing often competing considerations imply for the design and evaluation of childhood obesity interventions? Above all, we suggest, they call for a wide view of intervention effects, a view that is best obtained by taking account of the voices of those affected. As we argued in chapter 2, the primary aim of childhood obesity interventions should be to achieve tangible health improvements for children and to prevent poor health outcomes, while keeping in view other possible benefits, harms, and costs. This requires that we start from a broad understanding of the outcomes associated with childhood obesity interventions, so as to capture both positive and negative effects. To capture more fully the effects, both positive and negative, associated with an intervention, we must choose a wide range of outcome indicators. For example, in addition to information about weight changes associated with an intervention, we may want to include other measures, such as changes in self-esteem, body image, or disordered eating (see, e.g., Lumeng et al., 2006). Here we think it is particularly important to elicit parents' and, where appropriate, children's views on proposed or existing interventions. This is both because it may be difficult to identify relevant outcomes in advance, and also because the extent to which measures generate benefits or harms partly depends on how they are perceived by those affected.

Conclusions

Policy makers have become increasingly sensitive to the existence of social inequalities in health, and many governments and organizations have emphasized the importance of reducing such inequalities. Inequality is also a significant concern in the context of childhood obesity. As with most other health conditions, childhood obesity tends to be more pronounced among lower socioeconomic groups, ethnic minorities, and other disadvantaged groups, such as migrant families. The greater prevalence of childhood obesity among disadvantaged groups can exacerbate social inequalities in health and may also contribute to inequalities in other dimensions, such as education or income. Reducing or preventing childhood obesity among disadvantaged groups has been adopted as an explicit goal by many policy makers and can contribute to the reduction of social inequalities in health as well as inequalities in other domains. However, the design and evaluation of such strategies poses many challenges. To evaluate the full impact of particular interventions, it is crucial to develop a clearer understanding of both the benefits and harms to which interventions can lead, both to those who are the target of the intervention (e.g., children) and those who are affected indirectly (e.g., parents). As we suggested above, social research can help this process by identifying potential benefits and burdens associated with specific interventions and by providing information on barriers to participation for different groups. While it may turn out that interventions benefit worse-off groups on many dimensions, we may also find that there are difficult trade-offs to be made. Such trade-offs and compromises raise important questions about political priorities and the social distribution of responsibilities. As such they call for public debate and democratic decision making, including careful consideration of the views of those who are likely to be most affected.

5 STIGMA AND WEIGHT BIAS

IMPLICATIONS FOR CHILDHOOD OBESITY INTERVENTIONS

We have already referred to stigmatization as an important problem that needs to be taken into account as we think about childhood obesity and possible interventions to address it. The pervasive discrimination and stigmatization of overweight and obese adults is well documented in the literature. In this chapter, we focus on stigmatization and weight bias experienced by children and also consider questions of stigmatization as they affect parents.

The chapter begins with an overview of different approaches to stigma and related concepts before reviewing the empirical evidence on the stigmatization of obese and overweight children. The stigma that surrounds obesity has profound effects on children—primarily those who are overweight or obese but sometimes also those whose weight is classed as "normal." We discuss the implications of this problem for policy interventions that aim to prevent or reduce childhood obesity. In particular, we argue that considerations of stigmatization and its far-reaching effects should be explicitly integrated into the childhood obesity "agenda." We need both to take account of possible stigmatizing effects of particular interventions and adopt the reduction of weight bias as an important goal in its own right. As we have argued in earlier chapters, we must adopt a broader perspective that takes children's health and well-being as a primary goal, rather than being preoccupied by weight-related indicators such as BMI. We also reject the idea that the reduction of weight-based stigma could run counter to anti-obesity efforts: the notion that stigmatization could "motivate" weight loss and lead to health improvements is, to our mind, especially offensive and unhelpful. Despite our hesitation in this book to advocate particular priorities or solutions, the case against stigmatization strikes us as clear-cut: this is one part of the "war on obesity" that we would be better off without.

Conceptual Issues: Definitions of Stigma and Related Concepts

Many discussions of stigma start from Erving Goffman's *Stigma: Notes on the Management of Spoiled Identity* (1963). Goffman describes stigma as (evidence of) an attribute that marks an individual out as different from, and as less than, others. The person bearing such an attribute "is thus reduced in our minds from a whole and usual person to a tainted, discounted one" (p. 12). Familiar kinds of stigma include physical deformities, time spent imprisoned or in mental institutions, and membership of a particular ethnicity or religion. Central to stigma is that "the normals" (i.e., those not bearing stigmatizing attributes)[1] believe that

> the person with a stigma is not quite human. On this assumption we exercise varieties of discrimination, through which we effectively, if often unthinkingly, reduce his life chances. We construct a stigma theory, an ideology to explain his inferiority and account for the danger he represents, sometimes rationalizing an animosity based on other differences. (p. 15)

Goffman describes the experience of bearing stigmatizing attributes and its effects on individuals, as well as the tensions caused when individuals whose stigmatizing attributes are not immediately obvious try to manage others' knowledge of these features.

In a related analysis, Link and Phelan analyze stigma as the combination of six elements. First, stigma involves the identification and labeling of human difference; second, this difference is linked to undesirable characteristics ("stereotyping"); third, stigmatization allows for a separation between "them" (the group identified as different) and "us." Stigmatized individuals experience discrimination and loss of status (the fourth and fifth conditions). Finally, they regard as central to stigma that these processes are fueled by the exercise of power (Link & Phelan, 2006).

Other accounts, including those in the public health field, employ somewhat wider notions of stigma. Puhl and Latner (2007) define weight stigma as "negative weight-related attitudes and beliefs that are manifested

---

1. An important aspect of weight stigma is that those suffering from the stigma often seem to share the negative view that the "normals" have of them. We discuss the issue of "internalization" of weight stigma below.

by stereotypes, bias, rejection, and prejudice toward children and adolescents because they are obese or overweight" (p. 558). Their account of weight stigma also includes overt behaviors such as "verbal teasing (e.g., name calling, derogatory remarks, being made fun of), physical bullying (e.g., hitting, kicking, pushing, shoving), and relational victimization (e.g., social exclusion, being ignored or avoided, the target of rumors)" (Puhl & Latner, 2007, p. 558). Importantly, this definition includes both the holding of particular views or attitudes and the actions that express these attitudes. This definition is, in this sense, broader than Goffmann's but it strikes us as useful and appropriate to include these "external expressions" of stigma within our analysis.

For the purposes of this chapter, we adopt a perspective that is broader in another respect too. As we explain in more detail below, it has been suggested that some children regard as desirable body shapes that are *below* a healthy weight; among girls, particularly, even "normal weight" bodies may be regarded as undesirable. Thus, even normal weight children may be subject to weight-based teasing or stigmatization. It may also be that children fear becoming fat and its social consequences and engage in forms of food avoidance or disordered eating as a result. If we are concerned about the role of interventions with respect to weight-based stigmatization, we must therefore take into account its effects not just on overweight children but also on those whose weight counts as normal or even underweight.

Evidence of Stigmatization and Discrimination of Overweight and Obese Children

A substantial number of studies document weight bias and discriminatory behaviors against fatter children and adults in Western societies, including overweight people being bullied or avoided, discriminated against in hiring decisions, or being the subject of pejorative humor (MacLean et al., 2009). The acceptability of weight bias, compared to other forms of bias, is often noted in the literature. Stunkard and Sorenson (1993), for example, note that "now that prejudice against most formerly stigmatized groups has become unfashionable, if not illegal, one of the last acceptable forms of prejudice is that against obese persons" (p. 1387). This section discusses some of the empirical evidence on stigma and different kinds of weight bias experienced by (primarily, but not exclusively, overweight and obese) children.

Children—including children as young as three years of age (Harriger et al., 2010)—endorse thinness and exhibit weight bias; overweight and obese children thus find themselves exposed to weight bias from their peers. In a classic study by Richardson et al. (1961), children aged 10–11 years were asked to rank pictures of six children according to who they would most prefer to be friends with. Four of those pictures showed children with different disabilities (amputated hand, wheelchair, crutches, facial disfigurement). The remaining two pictures depicted children without disabilities, but one portrayed an obese child while the other showed a child of average weight. While the focus of Richardson et al.'s article is on disability, not weight, it is striking that the overweight child is generally ranked last. This study was replicated recently, finding that children were more strongly biased against the obese child than the children in the 1961 study (Latner & Stunkard, 2003).

In another study, nine-year-old girls were more likely to attribute negative traits to overweight people when asked to what extent they agreed with statements such as "fat people are smart" and "thin people are smart" for attributes such as happiness, laziness, or attractiveness (Davison & Birch, 2004). And in a further study, children aged seven–nine years were shown drawings of boys and girls with different body shapes and asked to rate each picture with respect to particular positive and negative traits (e.g., "kind," "funny," "lonely," "lazy," "ugly"). The drawings of thin children were viewed most favorably and those of overweight children least favorably (Kraig & Keel, 2001).

Weight-related teasing is also common among children, with one study suggesting that 45 percent of overweight children had experienced that kind of teasing (Haines et al., 2006; see also Haines [2010], for a general overview of the empirical literature on teasing). In a study by Neumark-Sztainer et al. (2002), 63.2 percent of obese adolescent girls (BMI ≥ 95th percentile) and 58.3 percent of obese boys reported being teased by their peers about their weight. One study found that obese and overweight adolescents were more socially isolated than their normal weight peers (Strauss & Pollack, 2003).

As we noted above, the effects of weight-based stigma may also be felt by children whose weight is classed as "normal." One study finds that, for girls, the desirable or "normal" body shape is thin rather than average-weight, and both normal weight and overweight are perceived negatively (Kraig & Keel, 2001); among girls, then, "the preference for thinness is so strong than even average weight is unacceptable" (Latner & Schwartz, 2005, p. 56). It may therefore be the case that even children whose weight is average or even below average are treated negatively by their peers.

It also appears to be the case that children are exposed to stigma and weight bias from educators and others whose duty it is to help them.[2] In a survey of 115 teachers, school nurses, and school social workers from high schools, 20–25 percent of respondents agreed that obese people were more emotional, less tidy, less likely to succeed at work, or more likely to have more family problems than non-obese people. About 25 percent agreed with the statement that "one of the worst things to happen to a person would be for him/her to become obese" (Neumark-Sztainer et al., 1999). Given the emphasis often put on physical education in schools as one way to address obesity, it is alarming to note that physical education teachers may exhibit even greater prejudice. A study with physical education students found that their implicit antifat bias was greater than for non-physical education students, and that this bias was stronger in students nearing the completion of their degree than in those who were just beginning their studies (O'Brien et al., 2006).

Finally, children may also experience weight bias from their own families, including their parents. In a study by Keery et al. (2005), 12 percent of middle school girls reported that their parents teased them about their weight, whereas Neumark-Sztainer et al. (2002) find that 47 percent of obese adolescent reported that they had been teased about their weight by family members (compared to 24 percent of average weight adolescent girls—itself a shocking figure); 34 percent of obese boys and 11 percent of average weight boys reported weight-related teasing by family members. One US study found that parents were less likely to fund their daughters' higher education if the daughter was overweight; further investigation suggested that this was the result of parental antifat prejudice (Crandall, 1995). The research suggests that weight bias and stigmatization is pervasive in children's lives.

Parents of Obese Children

The previous section sketched some of the forms and sources of weight stigma that children may experience in their everyday lives. In this section we briefly address two implications of this for parents.

First, as we have mentioned in chapters 2 and 3, this stigma places parents in a difficult position. Parents who are concerned about their children's

---

2. Regarding bias on the part of health care professionals, see the references given at the beginning of the section of this chapter titled, "Effects of Stigma on Individuals."

health and well-being need to be aware of the extent to which their children are subject to such stigmatization and how well they are coping with it. At the same time, they want to encourage their children to adopt a healthy diet and level of physical activity. Especially if their child is already overweight, or sees him- or herself as too heavy, they are likely to worry that such encouragement may reinforce, to their child's mind, the negative and destructive messages they are receiving from other children or from teachers and other adults. One of the researchers whose work we have already mentioned, Dianne Neumark-Sztainer (2005), has devoted an entire book targeted at parents who want to encourage appropriate diet and physical activity in their children, while being sensitive to the effects of weight stigma and the overemphasis on thinness that characterizes contemporary societies.

Second, weight stigma may extend not just to overweight children but also to their families. Parents of overweight and obese children may be the target of stigmatization themselves. In chapter 3 we criticized some of the simplistic rhetoric that attributes a key role to parental responsibility for rising rates of childhood obesity. Consider, for example, the suggestion that parents of very obese children may be charged with neglect or the children be placed under protective custody (Alexander et al., 2009; Cole & Kmietowicz, 2007; Murtagh & Ludwig, 2011). Despite the rarity of such extreme cases, this issue attracts frequent and disproportionate media discussion. Even when the aim is to keep charges of neglect distinct from moral judgments about parents (as suggested by Varness et al. [2009]), parents are quickly blamed when their child's weight is not within a "healthy" range. The relevant empirical evidence—suggesting the multitude of factors that contribute to obesity in children and reports that weight loss may be extremely difficult to achieve—is often neglected in these debates.

In a similar vein, Puhl and Latner (2007) are concerned that the pressure and negative judgments that parents of obese children are likely to feel could create their own problems. As already noted, stigma and discrimination may occur even within the family. Puhl and Latner hypothesize that parents may take out their frustration, anger, and guilt on their overweight child by adopting stigmatizing attitudes and behavior, such as making negative and critical comments toward their child. There is, however, little empirical investigation of the stigmatization of parents of obese children, or its effects within the family. Edmunds finds that parents' interactions with general practitioners sometimes lead them to feel guilty or blamed (Edmunds, 2005). A study by Hughes et al. (2010) found that low-income mothers often felt responsible for their children's overweight, in light of both genetic and behavioral explanations of the etiology of obesity in children:

> Many mothers—especially those who were overweight or obese—experienced tension because both explanations [i.e. those linking overweight to genetic factors and those regarding it as resulting from behavioral factors] could make them feel responsible and blamed for their children's weight. Mothers seemed to perceive that their children's weight status might reflect poorly on their parenting skills and, therefore, their identity as parents. This tension seemed greatest for those mothers who perceived that their children had inherited a tendency to be overweight. (p. 468)

The broader lack of evidence on this issue makes it difficult to assess the extent of the problem. We were unable to find any studies examining the stigmatization of parents of obese children, which strikes us as a serious omission. If we are concerned about how the experience of being the parent of an overweight or obese child is affected by interventions, then this is clearly an important area for research. As we argued in chapter 3 and consider further in chapter 6, one of the aims of interventions and other policies must be to support parents; measures that make parents feel anxious or guilty are invariably unfair and unlikely to have beneficial effects.

Effects of Stigma on Individuals

The general negative attitude toward overweight and obese individuals has far-reaching implications. For example, the public perception of obesity may affect the level of funding available for treatment of medical problems associated with obesity (Link & Phelan, 2006). Weight bias on the part of health professionals may mean that overweight patients receive lower-quality care than their average weight peers. (Such bias has been extensively documented, see Bertakis and Azari [2005]; Bocquier et al. [2005]; Hebl and Xu [2001]; Mold and Forbes [2011]; Pantenburg et al. [2012]; Puhl and Brownell [2001]). Stigmatization can also affect individuals' health and well-being. Stigma is often internalized and its messages can become part of a person's self-concept, which has been linked to lower quality of life, poor self-esteem, depression, unemployment, and poor health outcomes (Stuber et al., 2008). Children, it has been suggested, may be particularly vulnerable to such internalization

(Stuber et al., 2008). Further, stigmatization can contribute to significant health problems, such as depression, hypertension, coronary heart disease, and stroke (for a summary of the empirical evidence, see Major & O'Brien [2005]).

This section reviews some of the evidence available on the effects of stigma and related factors, such as teasing, specifically on children. There have been a number of reports of children and adolescents who committed suicide, largely because they were teased or bullied by their peers (Haines, 2010). In addition, there is evidence suggesting that stigma and related factors have a negative effect on health and well-being and may also influence important health behaviors.

Among children, the effects of weight-based teasing have been particularly well documented. Many studies have found that children who are teased about their weight have poorer psychological outcomes than those who are not teased (Haines, 2010; Keery et al., 2005). Specifically, teasing has been shown to lead to depressive symptoms, low self-esteem, body dissatisfaction, anger and anxiety, and suicidal ideation (see Eisenberg et al., 2006; Eisenberg et al., 2003; Iobst et al., 2009; Keery et al., 2005; Libbey et al., 2008; Lunner & Werthem, 2000). The research also suggests that these effects can be long-lasting, with teasing in the past affecting behavior far beyond the experience of teasing (Eisenberg et al., 2006).

In addition to the direct implications of stigma for health and psychological well-being, the experience of stigmatization may also affect individuals' health behaviors. Studies have found associations between weight teasing and bulimic behaviors (Keery et al., 2005), binge eating (Neumark-Sztainer et al., 2002), unhealthy weight control behaviors such as fasting and skipping meals (Neumark-Sztainer et al., 2002), or the use of laxatives, diet pills, and vomiting (Libbey et al., 2008).

It has also been suggested that stigma may contribute to obesity by increasing overweight children's fear of going out or being ridiculed while exercising (MacLean et al., 2009). For overweight adults, particularly women, evidence suggests that they are reluctant to participate in preventive health screening; for example, they are less likely to have pap smears and mammograms (Ferrante et al., 2007). While, to our knowledge, there have been no studies to determine whether similar effects can be found for overweight children, health educators need to be aware that focusing on children's weight in a critical manner may lead to similar avoidance of health professionals and preventive activities (O'Dea, 2010).

The empirical literature certainly paints a shocking picture of the extent and consequences of stigmatization for overweight and obese children. How significant are these consequences compared to the direct health effects of obesity? Activists argue that weight stigma, bias, and prejudice may in fact be causing more harm than health problems directly associated with obesity (see Oliver, 2006). Children are likely to be more sensitive to the effects of stigma than are adults (MacLean et al., 2009). With respect to the mental health of overweight children, it has been suggested that

> the negative psychological outcomes that have at times been connected with heavier body weight may be primarily the consequence of the negative reactions of others to excess weight. When statistically controlling for these negative reactions, the psychological outcomes often disappear. (Latner & Schwartz, 2005, p. 60; see also Eisenberg et al., 2003)

For adults, it has even been suggested that dissatisfaction with body weight (as measured by the difference between actual and desired BMI) is a better predictor of mental *and* physical health than BMI. As Puhl and Heuer (2010) summarize, "the high degree of psychological stress experienced by obese persons as a result of weight stigma contributes to the pathophysiology associated with obesity... many of the adverse biochemical changes that are associated with adiposity can also be caused by the psychological stress that accompanies the experience of frequent weight-based discrimination" (p. 1023, citing Muennig et al., 2008; Muennig, 2008). Since even very young children are exposed to stigma, and are very well aware of it as a daily reality, there is every reason to fear that similar mechanisms may apply in the case of children too.

Implications for Policy

How should the evidence on the effects of weight-based bias and stigma affect the kinds of policies we choose in preventing and treating childhood obesity? Three responses are discussed in this section. First, we argue that the idea that the stigmatization of certain behaviors can be an instrument in public health should be firmly rejected in the case of childhood obesity. Second, we argue that effects on stigmatization should be one of the factors assessed when particular interventions are evaluated, and interventions should be designed with this consideration in mind. Finally, we suggest that there is a substantial case for interventions that try to reduce stigma and/or its effects on children.

Stigma as an Instrument of Public Health?

In the public health field, experience with negative attitudes toward health conditions such as HIV/AIDS and mental illness have heightened awareness of the harms stigmatization creates for patients and their families. A range of policy initiatives has been developed with the specific aim of reducing stigma around such conditions. More recently, however, particularly in relation to smoking, there has been an increasing reliance on a strategy that uses stigmatization and "denormalization" of certain conditions and health behaviors in an attempt to bring about behavior change (Bayer & Stuber, 2006). Even though such a strategy may be problematic because of the burdens it imposes on those individuals whose behavior is stigmatized, it may be appropriate to use if its contribution to the health and well-being of the very people it burdens is sufficiently large (Bayer, 2008).

It might be suggested that a similar strategy could be adopted to address obesity: stigmatizing overweight and obesity as well as health behaviors, such as sedentary lifestyles or consumption of energy-dense foods, that contribute to it, could help motivate behavior change and further policy interventions. For example, an article by veteran bioethicist Dan Callahan (2013a) recently contended that we need

> to bring strong social pressure to bear on individuals, going beyond anodyne education and low-key exhortation. It will be imperative, first, to persuade them that they ought to want a good diet and exercise for themselves and for their neighbor and, second, that excessive weight and outright obesity are not socially acceptable any longer.... Obesity is in great part a reflection of the kind of culture we have, one that is permissive about how people take care of their bodies.... It will be necessary to make just about everyone strongly want to avoid being overweight and obese. (p. 37f)

Callahan (2013b) has subsequently explained that the printed text unfortunately was "left in some sentences from earlier draft versions—before I changed my mind, influenced by Rebecca Puhl—that ... stigma should be used on the obese and overweight" (p. 10). This was not before the printed views attracted a raft of criticism. As one writer bitingly put it, such a view seems "oblivious to the actual lived experiences of the people he would like ... to stigmatize. Callahan's whole idea is predicated on his own assumption that obese people either want to be fat, enjoy being fat, don't know they're fat, aren't willing not to be fat, or live in a world without any kind of media whatsoever and thus think everybody is fat" (O'Connor, 2013). As we have noted above, even children as young as three years of age (Harriger et al., 2010) endorse thinness and exhibit weight bias; there is nothing to suggest that they forget this bias as they grow up.

Even in his retraction, Callahan (2013b) restated his assumption that "many of the 108 million [Americans who attempted to lose weight in 2012] have been spurred by stigma—reflecting the possibility of making a choice about their weight" (p. 10). But the evidence that stigma—already amply present in almost every sphere of social life—actually leads to weight loss or health improvements is itself thin on the ground. While one study finds that greater experience of stigmatization may make patients more successful at weight loss (Latner et al., 2009), there is also evidence to suggest that the experience of stigma contributes to many behaviors that make overweight and obesity *more* likely: it can make overweight people less likely to exercise, encourage the adoption of dangerous and possibly counterproductive weight loss methods, and make them reluctant to seek medical assistance (Puhl & Heuer, 2010; Puhl & Latner, 2007). Thus, the pursuit of negative attitudes and stigmatization of obesity, or the behaviors that may contribute to it, is likely to be an unhelpful and counterproductive strategy. In addition, as we already highlighted in our introduction, media and advertising images in Western societies already do so much to promote thinness and stigmatize fatness that it is hard to imagine pushing this strategy any further than is effectively already the case.[3]

Evaluating the Effects of Interventions on Weight-based Stigma and Related Phenomena

A second policy concern related to the empirical evidence presented in this chapter pertains to the fact that anti-obesity interventions may *inadvertently* contribute to stigmatization. For example, O'Dea (2004) notes that

> the unintentional creation of body image and weight concerns, dieting, disordered eating and eating disorders is a probable outcome of childhood obesity prevention programs that focus on the 'problem' of overweight and refer to issues of weight control....Health education

---

3. The same point is made in many of the responses to Callahan's views printed in the issue of the *Hastings Centre Report* that also includes Callahan's own reply (2013b).

messages about overweight and weight control are likely to make young people feel worse about their bodies and themselves in general. (p. 260)

In a recent editorial, David Katz (2012) takes on the charge that anti-obesity interventions may contribute to the danger of disordered eating and unhealthy body image. He argues that as long as the goal is clearly children's health, rather than their weight per se, this risk can be minimized:

Our goal as health professionals should never be about weight, per se. It should be about health. If weight is too high to allow for health, weight should be lost. Not because of the importance of weight, per se, but because of what weight portends. If weight is too low to allow for health, weight should be gained, for just the same reason. Neither obesity, nor anorexia nervosa, is good for health. So if health is the destination, it should run away from both of these. (p. 415)

While we believe that Katz is right that the focus of health professionals' work should be on health rather than weight, he is too quick to dismiss the challenge to which he is responding. As we have mentioned above, it is difficult to communicate to a child that we are concerned about their health not their weight, especially when the child's weight is taken as a "marker" of health and a "gauge of progress" (Katz, 2012, p. 416). Moreover, as we have mentioned above, weight stigma is pervasive and affects health professionals just as much as—perhaps even more than—it does the general public. The fact that health professionals, whose job it is to communicate with patients about their health, are at least as prejudiced against overweight people means that it is unrealistic to assume that health professionals will not convey negative feelings they may have toward their overweight patients.

At the policy level, stigmatization should become a concern both in the design and evaluation of interventions. During the planning stages, those designing interventions might, for example, involve program recipients and elicit their responses to particular aspects of the intervention in order to avoid unintended and potentially harmful outcomes (O'Dea, 2004). For example, MacLean et al. (2010) suggest that to test for unintended effects of interventions, researchers could measure self-esteem before and after the intervention, for all weight categories. Of course, such evaluations require appropriate methodologies to measure different forms of stigmatization as well as its effects on individuals. Some researchers argue that better instruments need to be developed to do this (Puhl & Latner, 2007). Nonetheless, although precise measures are difficult to achieve and implement, some effects may be immediate and obvious and could be easily discovered by paying attention to the views of the children affected, or even, in some cases, simply by a little forethought:

> Dr. [Linda] Bacon tells the story of an overweight teenage girl whose high school was going through a "wellness campaign." Hallways were plastered with posters saying, "Prevent teenage obesity." After the posters went up, the girl said, schoolmates began taunting her in the halls, pointing at the obese girl on the posters and saying, "Look at the fat chick." (Brown, 2010)

Interventions to Reduce Stigma and Teasing Directly

In much of the literature on childhood obesity the psychological harm associated with obesity is presented or modeled as a *direct* consequence of obesity. As Cameron et al. (2006, p. xx) put it, "psychosocial problems, low self-esteem, and low self-image are the most common and immediate forms of morbidity associated with childhood obesity. These problems are pervasive in the families of obese children and increase as the child gets older" (see also Blacksher, 2008; Reilly et al., 2003). This approach makes weight loss the most plausible response to alleviate the psychological harms experienced by obese and overweight children. However, as mentioned earlier in this chapter, stigmatization of obesity is likely to be responsible for at least some of the negative outcomes in both mental and physical health among obese individuals. If many of these effects are due to people's attitudes toward obesity rather than obesity itself, challenging weight bias and stigmatization *directly* may lead to significant health benefits, as well as sparing much psychological distress.

A number of interventions have tried to address weight stigma and related factors among children. For example, Irving (2000) introduced a puppet program for primary school children to increase body size acceptance, healthy self-concept, and healthy attitudes about food and eating. Dealing with somewhat older children, Haines et al. (2006) developed an intervention called VIK (Very Important Kids) to prevent or reduce teasing as well as unhealthy weight control behaviors in children from fourth to sixth grades (with an average age of 10), many of them from low-income backgrounds. As part of the intervention, children produced a play in which students drew on their own experience of teasing to criticize this practice, and they also had a session with school staff to help them identify their attitudes toward weight and to learn about how to maintain a healthy body image. The results suggested that teasing had gone down as a result of the intervention, compared to the control group.[4]

However, researchers have also noted the lack of studies on interventions that seek to reduce weight stigma (Daníelsdóttir et al., 2010). For some, successful antistigma interventions must deal with some of the causes that feed negative attitudes toward weight. Rozin (1997) suggests that it is easier for moral judgments to come into play when there is confusion and limited understanding about particular health conditions, especially about the causes of those conditions. As we discussed in chapter 1, this clearly applies to obesity. Friedman (2004) argues that weight stigma is based, in part, on false assumptions about our ability to control our weight. The language of individual control and responsibility that is prevalent in public debates about obesity may therefore play an important role in stigmatization (Puhl & Heuer, 2010). With respect to children, one study concluded that when children blamed an obese model for being overweight, they were less likely to attribute positive traits to him or her (Iobst et al., 2009). This may suggest that promoting a better understanding of the causes of obesity and the limited control that individuals have over their weight could help combat weight stigma.

At the same time, a review by Daníelsdóttir et al. (2010) suggests that attempts to manipulate individuals' perspectives on the controllability of (over)weight have little effect on weight stigma. Recalling Goffman's comments about stigma (as discussed at the start of this chapter), it may be that a belief in controllability serves to *rationalize* dislike and prejudice, rather than itself leading to negative judgments. Daníelsdóttir et al. see more promise in interventions that seek to change social norms surrounding attitudes toward overweight and obese individuals. For example, in one study, messages about the social acceptability of particular attitudes influenced participants' willingness to condone or condemn a statement about weight bias—for example, "People should be able to tell jokes that make fun of obese people" or "People who discriminate against obese people should be punished" (Zitek & Hebl, 2007). While research findings remain inconclusive, then, it seems that both messages—that overweight cannot easily be controlled and that weight stigma is unacceptable—should play a role in attempts to reduce weight stigma.

---

4. See also chapter 9 on school-based interventions.

Conclusion

Stigmatization is a common experience for overweight and obese children and adults across different spheres of their lives. Even within their own families, children are often subject to negative attitudes regarding their weight. Apart from being unfair and cruel, the evidence suggests that these attitudes are very harmful to children who are exposed to them. While weight-related bias and stigmatization have only recently begun to attract significant research, studies suggest that this experience has far-reaching consequences, primarily in terms of negative effects on mental and physical health as well as on health-related behaviors.

From a policy perspective, these findings are extremely important. As we have emphasized throughout the previous chapters, it is crucial that we take a broad perspective when thinking about strategies to reduce obesity among children. Weight stigma must form part of this perspective: the effects of stigma on children's well-being and health are immediate and significant, and they deserve far greater attention than they have been getting so far. The current emphasis on weight as an indicator of health, illness, or risk of illness may have damaging and counterproductive consequences for children. It is therefore crucial to consider the ways in which particular interventions could exacerbate weight stigmatization and, more positively, explore the possibility that interventions that can successfully reduce weight stigma could make a crucial contribution to the health and well-being of children, be they overweight or not.

POLICY DOMAINS

CHILDHOOD OBESITY AND THE "OBESOGENIC ENVIRONMENT"

The environments in which people live are widely recognized as crucial in shaping a whole range of health outcomes. Over the last 150 years in developed countries, a series of environmental improvements—for example, in sanitation, food safety and distribution, and work safety standards—has accounted for the majority of improvements in life expectancy and levels of illness and injury (Centers for Disease Control and Prevention, 1999). A reverse but parallel point can be made regarding the characteristic diseases of modern Western societies: the common cancers, diabetes, and heart disease reflect an increase in chronic as opposed to communicable disease and are heavily influenced by our environments. Likewise, much of the current debate about chronic disease focuses on the role of the "social determinants of health" in contributing to poor health outcomes (e.g., Marmot & Wilkinson, 2003).

In a similar way, the environments in which most of us live are—for all their other benefits—now widely recognized as an important contributor to rising rates of obesity, and the term "obesogenic" has been coined to describe these environments. According to Swinburn and Egger (2002), "increasingly obesogenic environments are the predominant driving forces behind the escalating obesity epidemic and demand much more attention for research and action" (p. 297). The environments of developed societies are conducive to the development of overweight and obesity among individuals in two general respects. First, they encourage lifestyles that are largely sedentary rather than physically active: many occupations involve little, if any, significant physical activity during the day; most of us rely on cars and other forms of "inactive" transport to get to our place of work or other destinations; and leisure time activities are constrained by a range of factors, including concerns about personal safety, lack of attractive parks and green spaces, and financial constraints in accessing gyms and sports facilities. The second aspect of obesogenicity refers to characteristics of the environment that encourage the consumption of calories at a level that exceeds the energy expended. Again, many factors are involved, such as time constraints in buying and preparing fresh foods; the availability of energy-dense processed foods through fast-food restaurants, convenience stores, and supermarkets; marketing campaigns that promote the consumption of these foods; and large portion sizes in restaurants and for many processed foods and drinks.

Concerns about the obesogenic environment also apply to children. With respect to physical activity, many children now spend considerable time engaged in sedentary activities, such as watching TV. Many parents are concerned that it is unsafe for their children to walk or cycle to school and to play outside. A lack of parks and playgrounds may also contribute to low rates of physical activity among children. The food industry recognizes children as "future consumers" and actively mobilizes children's "pester power" to influence parents' purchasing decisions. By an overwhelming margin, the foods marketed to children are processed, energy-dense products that reflect intensive research on children's taste and consumption preferences.

Researchers and policy makers alike have sought to address these factors in an attempt to curb obesity rates among children. A number of high-profile interventions aim to alter these environmental factors in order to address childhood obesity. Measures to improve facilities for walking and cycling, to improve the availability of fresh fruits and vegetables, to increase the price of high calorie foods, to limit numbers of fast-food outlets, or to regulate marketing by food companies are among the many interventions that have been advocated as ways to make environments less obesogenic.

To focus on environments raises a series of public and policy questions. In this chapter, we consider a range of general issues facing policies that seek to reshape various aspects of the obesogenic environment. This chapter therefore provides the background to the analysis of specific policy issues in subsequent chapters: taxation and subsidization of particular foods, restrictions on food marketing, and school-based interventions. To the extent that we are concerned with particular intervention strategies in the present chapter, most of them are ones that relate to the physical environment, such as the "collective availability of sidewalks, parks, trails, recreational facilities, traffic safety, and other neighborhood characteristics that promote recreational PA [physical activity] as well as active transport to work, school, or errands" (Ferdinand et al., 2012, p. e7).

Questions around the obesogenic environment obviously connect with several themes already addressed in this book, and we would like to highlight two of these straightaway. First, questions of responsibility are crucial. In chapter 3, we raised the question of who should be regarded as responsible for childhood obesity and which duties different actors have to address it. Of particular concern in the present chapter will be the question of what duties local and national governments have when it comes to the obesogenic environment: What kind of environment should they provide or foster for children and their parents? We conclude this chapter by arguing that there is a strong case for governmental action to establish a reasonably healthy environment.

Second, questions of fairness and equality recur throughout this chapter. Disadvantaged families often find themselves in environments that are particularly obesogenic. They may have less access to healthy foods or must make longer commutes; multiple jobs or shift work may give them less time to prepare meals from scratch; there may be fewer recreational opportunities in their neighborhoods. At the same time, policy initiatives may not always reach these groups. As with other intervention strategies, the possibility of unequal access is an important concern when we are considering policies to tackle the obesogenic environment; at the same time, it may be that appropriate environmental policies could be of special benefit to families of lower socioeconomic status.

This chapter proceeds as follows. The first two sections raise some general questions that arise when obesity rates are linked to environments. First, we examine the term "obesogenic," the factors usually associated with it, and how it applies to children in particular. The host of factors that this term covers makes analysis and empirical investigation of the relative importance of *particular* aspects of the obesogenic environment difficult. Second, we consider some political issues raised when we make the environment our focus of attention. We argue that it is politically important to focus on shared environments, especially as a prompt to reconsider the status quo. The following section distinguishes between different ways of intervening in the obesogenic environment and discusses whether interventions should be thought of as removing opportunities or increasing them. The various environmental intervention strategies may have different advantages and disadvantages. Broadly, however, we argue that interventions can be in the interests of both children and their parents, and that it is unhelpful to assume that interventions to improve children's situation necessarily impose costs on, or restrict the liberties of, parents. The chapter concludes by emphasizing the key role of state actors in addressing obesogenic environments.

The Obesogenic Environment: What Is It and How Relevant Is It to Childhood Obesity?

The idea of the obesogenic environment has been gaining attention in the debate as a crucial ingredient in growing rates of obesity, both among adults and children. This section discusses the notion of the obesogenic environment and outlines what we know about its relative importance for childhood obesity. The concept of the obesogenic environment is very broad and includes a wide range of often very disparate factors. Furthermore, as with other areas, the evidence regarding the influence of the obesogenic environment in general—and that of specific factors in particular—is characterized by uncertainty. This naturally makes it much harder to recommend specific policies to change environmental factors in the confidence that these will improve childhood obesity rates.

Many discussions on the obesogenic environment and its role in rising obesity rates start from the definition of obesogenicity offered by Swinburn et al. Obesogenicity refers to "the sum of influences that the surroundings, opportunities or conditions of life have on promoting obesity in individuals or populations" (Swinburn et al., 1999, p. 564). Their analysis focuses on two major concerns: first, the degree to which an environment is conducive to sedentary lifestyles rather than a healthy level of physical activity; second, the degree to which it encourages or discourages the consumption of an amount of calories greater than energy expended. Different features of the environment can then act as barriers—or enablers—to healthier behaviors.

A very broad range of factors can be subsumed within the idea of the obesogenic environment. To facilitate analysis, Swinburn et al. propose two sets of distinctions. First, they suggest that we distinguish between micro- and macro-level environments. The micro-level includes particular settings in which people gather for different purposes, such as schools, neighborhoods, or workplaces. The macro-level is geographically diffuse and involves infrastructural factors or groups of industries and services that influence food and physical activity choices.

They also suggest a four-fold set of distinctions among relevant environmental factors. First, the *physical* environment captures food availability through, for example, restaurants, supermarkets, or vending machines. It also captures opportunities for physical activity. Factors that influence the use of active transport such as cycling and walking over inactive ones (e.g., escalators, lifts) include the availability of cycle and footpaths, public transport, and street lighting. Physical activity during leisure time is shaped by features of the physical environment such as availability of, and access to, green spaces, sports grounds, and parks. Second, *economic* features of the obesogenic environment refer to the cost of food and physical activity, which may be influenced by the use of subsidies, monetary incentives, or taxation schemes. Swinburn et al. also refer to *political* features of the obesogenic environment, which relate to formal as well as informal rules affecting food choices and physical activity, including, for example, food industry policies and regulations and policies relating to food marketing. Finally, Swinburn et al. identify *sociocultural* features of the environment. These features relate to norms, attitudes, and beliefs relevant to physical activity and food consumption. Such norms may be reflected, at the micro-level, for example, in the "ethos" of a school, neighborhood, or institution. At the macro-level, Swinburn et al. point to the media as an important factor shaping societal attitudes and values.

These distinctions are helpful partly because they show how broad a range of factors are bound up with the obesogenic environment—factors as wide-ranging as public transport facilities, density of fast food outlets, school canteens, advertising, and social norms surrounding physical activity and eating. Nonetheless, there may also be significant factors that are not readily captured within the categories mentioned. For example, concerns about personal safety—perhaps relating to perceptions of crime—may have an important influence on physical activity—and may be a particularly salient factor when it comes to childhood obesity. Studies suggest that, among parents, road and personal safety is a central concern in deciding whether children are allowed to play in certain locations (see, for example, Aarts et al., 2012; Carver et al., 2012). Other studies find associations between perceived neighborhood safety and obesity among children. For example, Lumeng et al. (2006) found that children whose parents perceived neighborhoods to be particularly unsafe were more than four times as likely to be obese than children whose parents perceived their neighborhoods as safe.

How does the obesogenic environment affect children, and which factors make environments more or less obesogenic from children's perspective? It is hard to ignore glaring changes in children's physical environment over recent decades: a significant portion of children's playtime is now spent in sedentary activities. Similarly, processed snack foods, often made to appeal specifically to children—for example, through images of well-known cartoon characters on packaging—have become near ubiquitous. It seems natural, therefore, to assume that these changes have played a significant role in the increases in childhood obesity rates we have been seeing across the developed world—and increasingly also in developing countries.

A number of studies have found correlations between environmental factors on the one hand and physical activity and diet on the other. Saelens et al. (2012), for example, find that for both children and parents, obesity rates were lowest in neighborhoods that were characterized by environments favorable to both healthy diet and physical activity (the former was captured in terms of proximity to supermarkets and low density of fast-food restaurants, the latter in terms of built environments conducive to walking and offering park access). At the same time, other authors caution that there is considerable uncertainty surrounding such research—not least, for the sorts of reasons we considered in chapter 1. Sallis and Glanz (2006) emphasize that it may be difficult to gauge from available evidence which factors of the built environment contribute to obesity among children, as most of the available studies have focused on adults. Similarly, a systematic review of quantitative research on the environmental influences on overweight and obesity in children and adolescents notes that "few consistent findings emerged" (Dunton et al., 2009, p. 399). Researchers have also expressed worries about the methods employed in empirical studies. Papas et al. (2007), for example, caution that studies tend to be cross-sectional and therefore do not allow for conclusions about causal connections between particular environmental factors and particular health outcomes. The use of inconsistent indices across studies—for example, of walkability—also reduces the comparability of the available evidence (Dunton et al., 2009). Nonetheless, it needs to be borne in mind that such difficulties are intrinsic to the subject matter—"walkability" represents a complex bundle of factors, and there is no straightforward way to measure, aggregate, and compare them all.[1]

Similarly, uncertainty exists around the effectiveness of particular intervention strategies, which makes it difficult to translate findings into concrete policy recommendations. Kirk et al. (2010) refer to the idea of the obesogenic environment as "a nebulous concept" and suggest that this complexity makes it difficult to identify which levels obesity prevention efforts should target (p. 110). It has also been noted that few successful strategies have emerged when it comes to environmental interventions targeted at children. Farley et al. (2007), for example, maintain that, "in spite of the recognition of environmental effects, few interventions have been developed that

---

1. Moreover, as we mention below, walkability means different things to different groups. The environmental factors necessary or desirable for young children to be physically active are quite different from those of adults or the old and infirm.

increased physical activity or reduced obesity in children by changing their environment" (p. 1625; see further Metcalf et al., 2012). Similarly, a review by Swinburn and Egger (2002) notes that interventions seemed to have effects of only modest magnitude on dietary behaviors.

Despite this uncertainty, researchers have argued that interventions that address obesogenic environmental factors are crucial in addressing (childhood) obesity. A recent piece in the *British Medical Journal*, for example, suggests that the "predominant driver [for obesity] is environmental, and changes to the environment will be essential if we are to tackle the current epidemic" (Wilding, 2012). Similarly, Sallis and Glantz (2006) note that, "given the urgency of the childhood obesity epidemic, we cannot wait for optimal evidence and must instead base actions on the best available evidence" (p. 101).

Many questions raised when advocating particular policy prescriptions on the basis of inconclusive evidence have been discussed in chapters 1 and 2. Subsequent chapters will address policies and concerns around specific elements of the obesogenic environment: chapter 7 is concerned with policies to influence food prices, chapter 8 addresses marketing of unhealthy foods to children, while chapter 9 concerns the role of schools in addressing obesity. In the remainder of this chapter, our focus is on the broader question, the answer to which will also shape our responses to more specific policy issues: What are the concerns and particular advantages of policies that seek to redress the obesogenicity of the environment in which children and parents live? First, however, we would like to comment on the importance of framing these questions in terms of *environments*.

Framing the Issues: Environments as a Focus of Concern

To suggest that contemporary environments are problematic—from the point of view of childhood obesity or other concerns—is to make an important political move, just as the opposite tendency to focus on individual behavior also has a political dimension. These political aspects may not always be obvious and are therefore worth highlighting directly.

The sociologist C. Wright Mills (2000) once spoke of the need "to translate personal troubles into public issues," pointing out that "many personal troubles cannot be solved merely as troubles, but must be understood in terms of public issues" (p. 187). His point was that many people's lives are disturbed and disrupted in different ways—by discrimination, ill-health, poverty, and so on—and these problems are not merely personal ones. This is to oppose a common line of thought, which looks at such matters as personal or even private, without social and political dimensions: although charity may sometimes represent an appropriate response to some of these ills, there is no call for a public response. This sort of individualizing tendency has been a marked feature of public and political discourses in the United States, and to a lesser extent in some other countries such as the United Kingdom and Australia. Under the banner of personal responsibility and individual choice, strong claims are made about which issues merit collective action or state intervention—and which issues do not. These claims have been quite influential—although much depends on how questions are framed. American respondents tend to be quite willing to endorse such an approach to childhood obesity:

> Only 18% of Americans identify external factors (exposure to junk food, lack of safe places for children to play, and limited availability of healthy foods in some neighborhoods) as the biggest causes of childhood obesity, whereas 64% identify personal factors (overeating, lack of exercise, and watching too much television) as the biggest causes. (Barry et al., 2012, p. 389; citing Bleich & Blendon, 2011)

Against this background, to highlight structural features of the environment that shape the lives of many people represents an invitation to reframe the issues. The "personal troubles" facing children and parents—be they discrimination and bullying, or factors conducing to obesity and poor future health—are translated into public issues—such as the prevalence and acceptability of antifat prejudice, or the obesogenic environment.

So far, this does not yet involve any claims about responsibilities to shape or reshape that environment. Nor does it imply that altering environments will necessarily be the most effective way to address obesity—perhaps changes in individual behaviors would be more effective or might be more easily achieved. Nonetheless, it does at least raise the questions: What public or environmental factors have led to higher rates of obesity and can they be meaningfully addressed? To raise the environment as a public issue also invites two further questions that we already emphasized in the book's introduction. The first concerns priorities: How serious an issue is obesity, relative to the other problems and costs that are involved in our environments, and the opportunities and advantages that those environments supply? The second concerns responsibility: Who should have the responsibility to reach decisions about priorities and the power to intervene or reshape our environments in accordance with those judgments? How to balance all the different things that we want from our environments, how to balance the differing needs or desires of different parties, and how to act on the resulting judgments—all are crucial political questions.

Plainly, they are also questions without simple answers. One reason for this is that many of the factors that conduce to obesity also provide all sorts of benefits. It may yet be the case—to give an example that we mentioned at the start of chapter 1—that "as a result of the substantial rise in the prevalence of obesity…life expectancy at birth and at older ages could level off or even decline within the first half of this century" (Olshansky et al., 2005, p. 1142). Nevertheless, the fact remains that rates of life expectancy in modern Western societies are unprecedented. As we mentioned at the beginning of this chapter, this largely owes to environmental factors such as the easy availability of safe foodstuffs, the safe heating of our homes and workplaces, and the reduced need for strenuous or risky physical activity. Even when they do not make us healthier, comfort and convenience are things most of us still value highly. As we have stressed already, it is no simple matter to decide the relative priority of these different goods or the best arrangements for balancing them against one another. Nevertheless, there are reasons to think that we have not struck an ideal balance—not least, given how quickly rates of obesity have increased in most Western societies.

Another reason for the lack of simple answers lies in the complexity of our social divisions of responsibility. Western societies uphold extensive private rights alongside significant collective achievements—the plenty, security, and convenience already mentioned. Again, it is no simple matter to say what powers governments should assume or how governments (or other actors) should try to alter our environments. Since we are often wary of state power to reshape our private—or public—lives, and since the arrangements are already so complex, we may feel particularly reluctant to endorse state intervention, even where the state is the only actor with the power to substantially alter less desirable features of our environments.

Clearly, there are many problems raised by the environments and infrastructures of modern developed societies. Apart from problems of obesity, we mention just two: sustainability and equality. We have already raised questions of equality and social justice in chapter 4 and will mention below some ways in which a focus on obesogenic environments might complement this concern. The question of sustainability goes beyond our scope in this book, but we do think it is useful to highlight two ways in which questions of sustainability intersect with our concerns here. First, and very briefly, moves to combat, for example, unsustainable reliance on carbon-based energy may also alter how obesogenic our environment is. Measures to reduce car use, to create more efficient public transport systems, and to increase "active transport" (walking and cycling) can obviously promote sustainability and play a role in preventing obesity. Such overlaps need to be considered on a case-by-case basis. They are part of what we had in mind in chapter 2, in arguing that public policy needs to address many priorities simultaneously.

Second, there are some interesting ways in which the environments of modern Western societies invite us to idealize their workings and effects. These have posed grave problems for public appreciation of just how serious are the multiple crises of sustainability that we face. More generally, they tend to make otherwise desirable changes to our environments seem more challenging and costly than they would actually be—whether one thinks of measures to prevent obesity, address social justice, promote sustainability, or many other issues besides. In other words, it is not just reluctance to sanction greater (or different forms of) state intervention that can discourage moves to address obesogenic environments. We may also be reluctant because important factors lead us to view our current environments less than realistically—that is, to idealize them and ignore their costs, risks, and inconveniences.

To indicate what we have in mind, consider how the private car figures in our everyday awareness. This is not just an object of need or convenience or comfort. It is also socially invested with ideals of freedom, autonomy, and empowerment. Those ideals are continually massaged by advertisers and media representations. Images of "the open road" seem to have a life of their own, floating free of the more frustrating and complicated daily reality: traffic jams, expenses, breakdowns and repairs, the harried pursuit of errands that seem compulsory to any parent with a car—not to mention the less visible costs in pollution, children's freedom to play, road injuries, and public spending on roads.[2] If we could keep those harsher realities in mind, we might

---

2. There is also an individual as opposed to collective dimension to this problem. However much a person may be aware of problems in our reliance on the private car, the structure of our environments—both the physical layout of cities and suburbs in terms of roads and facilities, as well as shared provisions such as public transport—may make it very hard to manage without a car. However, our immediate point concerns a widespread tendency (for individuals, as well as in public debates) not to acknowledge the costs and risks bound up with our reliance on the car—a tendency that makes it much harder to take collective action to reduce our dependence upon it.

find it easier to strike a balance that does justice to all the concerns in play—including our children's health.

The wider issue we want to highlight is a selectivity in attention that affects food and consumption patterns as much as transport systems. Most of us never see the production processes behind the food and other goods we consume, and we see very little of how waste products—of both production and consumption—are dealt with.[3] By and large, what we see and pay attention to are the things we use and consume, just as they appear in advertisements, shops, and homes. This may sound innocent and is certainly something we take for granted. But it also poses significant risks and costs, because it insulates us from underlying realities and systematic effects: we perceive private consumer goods and personal opportunities, rather than public costs and environmental limits.

More than this, our perceptions are often idealizing or aspirational. As the example of the private car was meant to suggest, our relationships to the food, drink, and other goods we buy are mediated by carefully crafted advertisements, clever branding, and escapist entertainment: bucolic farms, open roads, prosperous suburban homes untouched by financial worry and other life-disrupting stresses. For those who are healthy and well-off, these pictures may not be so distant from reality, though they still obscure more than they reveal. For the worse-off, they are tantalizing visions of what might be: thus many brands trade on providing a small taste of a glossy and otherwise unobtainable reality. This veneer of idealization and aspiration makes it harder to engage with the less pleasant and more ambivalent realities.

The same veneer also obscures problems of choice and power. To a consumer, what is most obvious is the freedom and choice afforded by the many goods on offer. This will be less true for parents struggling to feed and clothe their family on a limited budget—but the tantalizing possibility of greater choice always remains in sight. What remains hidden, however, are two things. Obviously, we do not see alternatives that are not offered. For example, unless one has lived in a city with lively produce markets—the wonderful food markets of Barcelona, for example, distributed in neighborhoods across the city—one might hardly consider the possibility of cheaply and conveniently buying

---

3. This point is made very vividly by Annie Leonard in her now-famous video, *The Story of Stuff*, available via her project website www.storyofstuff.org; see also her subsequent book (2010). Or compare the novelty of the film *Toy Story 3* (Unkrich, 2010) in depicting the usual fate of consumer goods—the municipal rubbish dump. The enormous quantities of refuse generated by our societies are something that almost none of us have to see or think about, although they are essential to modern (sub)urban life.

a vast range of foods anywhere but in a supermarket. The many possibilities for reorganizing food systems and urban environments only become visible when we compare different societies—and even then, other possibilities remain mere ideas or yet to be imagined. Equally, we do not see how the terms of our choices are set. Why is it so easy to find a can of Coke or cellophane-wrapped muffin, and so hard to find a really tasty apple? Why do supermarkets dominate food retailing in most countries, and how can they sell many foods so cheaply? Large questions of power and profit lurk behind such questions. But for the most part they remain abstract, since there is not much pressure to ask them. The question that faces us most often is whether to buy one item rather than another.

Neither of these points is especially sinister or surprising. We have created systems that sustain themselves partly by marketing their benefits to us. Some of those benefits are real, but some of them are partly imaginary— the images of advertisers and the aspirations by consumers. Moreover, every reality is much more present to us—more realistic, one might say, and also more powerful—than the endless hypothetical alternatives. The problem we are highlighting is that this equips us quite badly for considering and pursuing alternative arrangements. This matters because food, consumption, and transport systems are such central factors of our obesogenic environments. Any attempt to alter these is bound to run into not just the benefits they provide, but also the ways in which we *perceive* those benefits. Were we able to keep all the costs of these systems firmly in mind—some of which are mere daily irritations (perhaps not even "personal troubles"), while others are much more serious and systematic ("public issues" of the first order)— attempts to change them would seem much more attractive.

Intervening in the Environment: Normative Considerations

Despite the politics implicit in emphasizing the obesogenic *environment*, policies that target it are often seen as less problematic than those that focus on individual behaviors, from an ethical point of view. Nonetheless, such strategies do raise distinctive normative issues, which we explore in this section.

Note first that when it comes to policies that seek to reduce the obesogenicity of the environment in which we live, two broad strategies can be distinguished. On the one hand, many policies have focused on *removing* options that are conducive to sedentary lifestyles or overconsumption of food. For example, policies that seek to ban fast-food outlets around schools

(Campbell, 2010) or in particular neighborhoods (Sturm & Cohen, 2009) fall into this category, as do the recent efforts of New York City mayor Michael Bloomberg to ban large-size sugar-sweetened soft drinks (Grynbaum, 2012). On the other hand, policies may seek to *add* healthier options or to make such options more attractive to individuals. Interventions that enhance or provide green spaces to encourage physical activity, for example, and those that seek to increase the availability of fresh produce in inner-city neighborhoods will fall into this second category.

A possible third category is that of so-called nudges or libertarian paternalism, which is receiving increasing attention in public health contexts (Ménard, 2010; Sunstein & Thaler, 2008), including obesity (Womack, 2012). "Nudges" involve small, often imperceptible changes in the way different options are presented to individuals so as to make healthy choices more likely. There have been some studies that have explored the possibility of using this approach in the context of childhood obesity. For example, Hanks et al. (2012) found that altering the arrangement of foods in school cafeterias could lead to greater consumption of healthier foods among children.[4]

In practice, of course, particular interventions may combine aspects from more than one of these categories. For example, a school-based initiative may reduce the availability of sweetened soft drinks through vending machines (or ban such drinks completely) while providing water fountains in corridors or making water more prominent in the dining hall. Similarly, adding new cycle routes may reduce the amount of space for car traffic and be implemented in such a way as to make the option of cycling more prominent in people's minds.

What, then, are the normative issues raised by interventions that focus on the obesogenic environment? We first consider the idea that environmental interventions may be paternalist and consider how this charge relates to parents' situation and responsibilities. While stressing the shared interests that parents and children may have in environmental interventions, we also note that adults and children may have rather different needs of their environments. We then consider how environmental policies relate to questions of equality, and finally, to questions of stigmatization.

Paternalism and the Interests of Parents and Children

The most prominent issue around environmental interventions concerns "paternalism." Paternalism describes interventions that restrict individuals'

---

4. For a critical response to the libertarian paternalist approach, see Hausman and Welch (2010).

liberties so as to increase their well-being (Dworkin, 2010; Nys, 2008) or to make it more likely that they will make choices that are conducive to their health. The charge of paternalism can arise when a policy removes options, when it requires people to pay (through taxation) for new options or public facilities, or (with "libertarian paternalism") when policies alter how choices are framed. There have been heated debates about the paternalism of public health interventions at all these levels. But although the charge of paternalism is often treated as a knock-down argument against a policy, some commentators have argued that certain paternalist interventions may be permissible, or even required (de Marneffe, 2006; Wilson, 2011). We discuss this point in more detail in chapter 7 when considering whether policies to tax or subsidize particular foods and drinks would be paternalist.

However, for obvious reasons, the term "paternalism" is not especially helpful in getting to grips with policies aimed at children's health. No doubt, interfering with children's activities and choices for their benefit may well be paternalist. But the root of the word "paternalism"—that is, in fatherhood or more generally, parenting—shows straightaway how inept it would be to criticize policies affecting children's lives from this point of view: given children's limited capacity for choice, paternalism is required in many situations (Scarre, 1980). This is not to deny that there may be good reasons for not restricting children's choices in particular contexts—precisely *because* "choosing" is a crucial skill that we want children to learn. This issue, and its implications for the childhood obesity debate, is discussed in chapter 9, where we consider the ethical issues surrounding school-based obesity interventions.

Nonetheless, even if it is not in itself problematic to restrict children's choices, many interventions that aim to reduce childhood obesity may affect what *parents* can do for their children or restrict the options available to them. For example, some interventions have targeted the foods that children are allowed to bring to school for snacks, lunches, and parties—with clear implications for what parents may provide. Another dramatic example was a UK school policy that prevented children leaving school grounds at lunchtime and hence from going to fast-food outlets. Notoriously, parents who disagreed with the policy were shown on television passing fish and chips through school fences (Anonymous, 2006). Or in the name of safety—rather than obesity prevention!—schools have often stipulated that children may not walk or cycle to school, leaving many parents with little option but to drive their children to school. Such policies are not, strictly speaking, paternalist because these restrictions are meant to benefit third parties (the children) rather than those whose liberties are restricted. Nonetheless, such policies attract suspicions of "overreach" and undue interference in parental choice and family life.

The resulting conflicts between schools', parents', and children's interests naturally attract media attention.[5] They also tend to highlight the negative role that parents can play and hence may encourage policies that restrict parents' freedom of action. Even where there are genuine conflicts, however, there are reasons to hesitate before endorsing restrictive policies. Where policies interfere with parents' ability to shape important aspects of their children's lives, they run counter to parental interests. Brighouse and Swift (2006), for example, argue that in addition to being charged with the responsibility for their child's well-being and development, parents also have an interest in being in this kind of relationship, in developing flourishing relationships with their children, and, to this end, shaping various aspects of their children's lives. Such parental interests should form part of our assessment of policies that restrict parental freedom of action, even if this consideration is often outweighed by a legitimate interest in ensuring children's health and well-being. There is also the fact that environmental policies are bound to affect all the children (and perhaps adults) in a particular area or school. Even if most parents welcome the policy, it is likely that some parents will be less convinced. In every case, however, we suggest that it is important to understand why parents may disagree with a measure, not only because they are the people who know their child best and because their cooperation is so often essential for measures to achieve the intended benefits, but also because their role as parents gives them rights that we have reason to accommodate.

More broadly, however, framing the issues in terms of children's interests as against parental liberties is not especially helpful. This is because it obscures how policies aimed at the obesogenic environment can support both parents and children and the importance of *empowering* parents to fulfill their responsibilities. As Brighouse and Swift (2006) put it, "much of the value of parenting comes precisely from being able to look after children's interests well, being there to give them what they need to develop into the kind of people it is good for them to become" (p. 107). Given that parents generally want their children to be healthy, parents' and children's interests are closely intertwined. The obesogenic environment often interferes with the actions that parents would like to take on behalf of their children. For example, as

---

5. Compare the amount of publicity and discussion devoted to cases where obese children have been removed from their families (as mentioned briefly in chapter 3).

we discuss in chapter 8, the food industry recognizes that even though small children rarely make their own food purchase decisions, their "pester power" can be harnessed to powerful effect. Parents who aim to reduce the amount of processed food their children consume may well find it difficult to insist on a healthy diet when their children repeatedly request cleverly engineered and marketed foods that have little to recommend them in nutritional terms.

The point about shared interests can also be framed in terms of empowering parents to fulfill their responsibilities. As we argued in chapter 3, when we consider any social role, it is vital that the demands it makes can be met by the people who will occupy that role. This is especially true when the role is as important as that of raising children. The obesogenic environment is problematic not only because of its negative effects on children's health and well-being, but also because it interferes with parents' ability to look after their children. (In the same way, as we already mentioned in chapters 3 and 5, an environment that involves systematic discrimination against fatter children makes it harder for parents to fulfill their tasks.) Environmental and structural policies can actively promote parents' ability to fulfill their responsibilities.

Having stressed how parents and children have a shared interest in many environmental interventions, we should also recognize that the needs of adults and children may come apart. For example, when we think of how conducive physical environments are to physical activity, this varies considerably depending on which age group we have in mind. As Davison and Lawson (2006) note:

> One cannot assume that associations between the physical environment and physical activity among adults are applicable to children.... In contrast to adults, [children] spend large parts of their day at school, have considerable time for recreation, are more likely to accumulate physical activity through play, are not able to drive, and are subject to restrictions placed on them by adults. (p. 2)[6]

This means that it is important to give specific attention to children's needs when, for example, planning or redesigning urban environments. This may sometimes involve trade-offs—depending on the particular constraints of an environment or planning rules, walkability may have to be sacrificed for "playability," or vice versa. However, as we have stressed, multiple goals and

---

6. See also Buck et al. (2011). Adolescents' needs may be different again: see also De Meester et al. (2012); Van Dyck et al. (2013).

constraints are a basic fact of life. As such, they tend to be most problematic when they are ignored—for example, when it is assumed that adults' and children's interests must be identical—than when we face the resulting complexities head-on.

Equality

The desire to address inequality may motivate environmental policies, but it may generate concerns too. On the face of it, environmental policies are attractive because they can reach a broad population and provide a range of benefits nonselectively. Importantly, these benefits can go far beyond individuals struggling with obesity or overweight: the factors that make the environments in which we live "obesogenic" are problematic for many people, even if they do not cause every person to become obese. As we have emphasized before, insufficient physical activity and poor nutrition are independent risk factors for a number of health conditions. Policies that help address these factors and support individuals in making healthy decisions can, therefore, have far-reaching benefits. Nonetheless, some of the concerns raised in chapter 4— that interventions may exacerbate inequalities—also come into play when we are assessing policies that seek to address the obesogenic environment.

Environmental strategies can, it is sometimes argued, be beneficial for disadvantaged groups that are often considered "hard to reach"—for example, low-income groups, ethnic minorities, or those with low educational levels (Swinburn et al., 1999). Moreover, policies can be specifically targeted to address problems faced by disadvantaged groups. We know that many aspects of the obesogenic environment are particularly salient for disadvantaged groups. For example, people on low incomes may find it harder to pay for gym memberships or physically active leisure activities for their children; they are more likely to have to rely on freely available opportunities for physical activity—such as parks and green spaces or playgrounds for their children—which are generally harder to find in low-income neighborhoods. Addressing such disparities through policies that improve these obesogenic factors could therefore help address inequalities in obesity rates and be of particular benefit for low-income families. As Swinburn and Egger (2002) maintain, "environmental interventions can not only reach populations with poor health outcomes but they can be differentially targeted to them, such as improving bus services, school food programs, and active recreation amenities in poorer areas" (p. 293). If successful, such interventions can therefore help address inequalities in the distribution of obesity across social groups.

Matters may be more complex in practice, however. Policies that enhance opportunities for physical activity and healthy nutrition do not, in themselves, ensure that such opportunities will in fact be taken up by individuals and families. In chapter 4 we discussed the concern that unequal uptake of public health initiatives may be counterproductive from the perspective of equality (see also Lorenc et al., 2013, for a systematic review of available evidence on this question). In other areas of public health, we have seen that it is primarily better-off groups that take advantage of available opportunities and that they benefit to a greater extent from public health campaigns. In the smoking context, for example, media campaigns have been found to be less effective with less educated groups (Niederdeppe et al., 2008). While there remains controversy and uncertainty regarding the specific causes of such disparities, a plausible overall explanation would simply run as follows: People who are better off tend to have more opportunities and more control over their lives, and so are better able to take up new opportunities or to act on information and advice.

Those designing intervention strategies have, of course, paid attention to problems around uptake of available resources and proposed possible solutions to this issue. Dunton et al. (2009), for example, suggest that the weak association between neighborhood characteristics, such as the availability of recreational facilities and parks, and childhood obesity outcomes may be the result of poor uptake. They caution, therefore, that environmental policies may have to be accompanied by outreach and educational activities.

However, this concern may be reduced in the case of policies that *restrict* opportunities for unhealthy choices. If we are increasing the availability of healthy options, there is scope for unequal uptake and hence increasing inequalities; when we remove unhealthy options, however, the scope for individuals to forego particular benefits is removed. For example, while the possibility of unequal uptake remains when we add fruit juices and water to the sweetened drinks available in school vending machines, removing sugar-sweetened beverages entirely means that *no* student has access to these through school vending machines. While interventions that add healthy options are often considered less problematic than those that remove unhealthy options, the latter may have advantages with respect to concerns about equality. However, as we now discuss, concerns about stigmatization may arise where restrictions are targeted or have differential effects on different communities.

Stigmatization

A further possible advantage of interventions that target children's physical environment is that they may be less likely than other kinds of interventions to carry problematic messages about body size. Hence they may avoid contributing to the stigmatization of overweight and obese children. As we stressed in chapter 5, countering this stigmatization should be a central consideration when it comes to efforts to reduce childhood obesity. Compared to strategies aimed directly at individuals, policies that seek to address the obesogenic environment are arguably less likely to carry messages of personal blame because they rely on the (implicit or explicit) assumption that environmental factors are contributing to obesity rates. Environmental policies that enhance the options available, or shift the balance in favor of walking and cycling, are most easily framed in terms of the causal role of environmental factors. For example, to make the case for increasing the availability of green spaces or lowering the price of fresh produce, we can argue that urban environments and high food prices create significant barriers for individuals who want to exercise or eat nutritious food.

However, when policies target particular areas or groups, or affect different communities differently, they may be perceived as stigmatizing—if not of overweight and obese people, then of the communities affected. As we emphasized above, disadvantaged groups often live in particularly obesogenic environments. It therefore seems natural to call for policies that seek to address these disadvantages. As an example, consider the controversial decision of the Los Angeles city council to restrict the opening of new fast-food restaurants in southern parts of the city, many of which are low-income and ethnic minority communities. The city council was careful to frame this move in terms of concerns about high obesity rates and as a response to the overconcentration of fast-food restaurants in these neighborhoods and the absence of restaurants and grocery stores offering healthier fare (Bernstein, 2010; Perry, 2007; Sturm & Cohen, 2009; Vick, 2008). Proponents of the policy emphasized that South LA had a much higher concentration of fast-food outlets than wealthier parts of the city and that the restrictions could help bring healthier food options into the area.[7]

Nonetheless, such a policy can be framed rather differently. Critics described it in terms of "local leaders across America seeking to impose a

---

7. Both of these points, however, were contested by critics (Sturm & Cohen, 2009).

healthier lifestyle on residents to counter soaring obesity rates" (Sherwell, 2008) and as "depicting poor people, like children, as less capable of free choice" (Saletan, 2008). An important part of the concern is that the initiative targeted low-income, ethnic minority communities. If initiatives such as these are taken to imply that the populations they target cannot be relied on to resist unhealthy food options, then such policies may well be seen to carry stigmatizing messages about poor people or those from ethnic minorities as less able to resist highly palatable foods and needing additional governmental intervention to make healthy choices.[8]

This is not to deny, of course, that structural and environmental policies may well be appropriate strategies to adopt, or that it may be appropriate to target them at areas or communities worst affected. However, these policies may carry—or be seen to carry—problematic messages. The more general point highlighted by such contestable examples is that it is rarely easy to address many different factors and concerns in complex settings. The difficulties involved call for reflection and debate on a case-by-case basis, with special attention to the views of groups or communities that are targeted or most affected.

Conclusion

It is clear that many changes in our physical, social, and economic environments are conducive to obesity. As a result, the idea of the obesogenic environment has been gaining momentum in policy debates about childhood obesity. In this chapter, we have outlined some of the issues surrounding the notion of "obesogenicity" and discussed the politics involved in highlighting "environments." We have also explored some of the normative issues around environmental strategies. Although commentators often assume that structural policies raise fewer ethical issues than marketing campaigns and interventions aimed at individual behaviors, they are not without issues.

Nonetheless, despite these problems—not to mention the allegedly "nebulous" (Kirk et al., 2010, p. 110) character of the idea—we have argued that focusing on obesogenic environments is politically valuable. It represents an important counter to individualizing tendencies that suggest that each person

---

8. Compare also the example of prohibiting the use of food stamps to purchase sweetened drinks, as discussed in chapter 4.

or family is responsible for their own choices. In blunter terms, such views simply mean that people should be left to fend for themselves as best they can. But the fact remains that powerful environmental factors set the terms against which we make our choices and determine the consequences of those choices. In particular, parents have only limited control over many aspects of their children's environment, their activity levels, and their diet. Parents who seek to encourage a healthy lifestyle in their children often find their efforts frustrated. This is especially true, we have suggested, for disadvantaged families and should add urgency to calls for policy changes that can make our environments more conducive to health.

Unless we want to leave parents and children exposed to an environment that sometimes fails to support children's healthy development, therefore, we need to locate actors who can bear the responsibility to alter those environments. Realistically (as we explore in the next two chapters), the key bodies here are states and local governments. Only states can take responsibility for public spaces, urban planning, and transport systems—roads, pavements, cycling routes, parks, and the rest. Only states can set the rules by which food markets operate. As we argue in chapter 7, their tax structures, subsidy schemes, regulations, and infrastructures play an important role in affecting food prices and availability. As we discuss in chapter 8, only states can alter the regulatory framework under which companies operate and prevent corporate actors from having an undue and unhealthy influence on children's lives. As we consider in chapter 9, schools—whose actions are more or less closely tied to state policies in different jurisdictions—may also play some role at very local levels.

In saying this, we do not mean to rule out the role of various nongovernmental organizations, such as parents' and neighborhood associations, which might well take an interest in the questions here. Some measures to alter local environments clearly lie within the grasp of parents (especially better-off parents) and community groups or organizations (especially in communities with higher levels of social capital). Their actions can also make an important difference to policy making and implementation. Indeed, if states and local governments are to act, they need the support and encouragement of their citizens. Nonetheless, the obesogenic environment represents a valuable way of framing a public issue, because it highlights the critical role of government and exposes structural problems covered over by some common ways of imagining and idealizing our societies. It remains a matter for public debate to settle the priority that ought to be given to addressing the obesogenic environment, relative to the many other issues facing our societies such as sustainability, inequality, and the lower status of many groups and communities. Likewise, public debate is needed to find ways of addressing those issues alongside one another and deciding who should implement these. Nonetheless, we would argue, public solutions and state action are clearly called for.

7 PRICE POLICIES AS STRATEGIES FOR OBESITY PREVENTION

In chapter 6, we discussed the idea of the "obesogenic environment" as a way of approaching childhood obesity. Despite the inevitably open-ended nature of this concept, we argued that it is helpful for thinking about the policy issues around childhood obesity. Rather than seeing obesity as a "personal trouble," it draws our attention to environmental or structural factors. Increasing childhood obesity rates thus become a "public issue" whose importance and implications for policy need to be debated and acted on. In this chapter, we turn our attention to one of the key environmental factors: the price and availability of food and drinks, especially sugar-sweetened ones.

Relative to other prices and income, food prices have declined over the past several decades. However, price changes have not been consistent across the board. Fresh fruit and vegetables have in fact become more expensive, while sugars, sweets, and soft drinks have become relatively cheaper (Figure 7.1). Decreases in price have also been seen for fats and oils and meat products (Finkelstein & Zuckerman, 2008, p. 20f; Leonhardt, 2009; Putnam et al., 2003, p. 15). All these foodstuffs tend to be more energy dense—that is, they contain more calories for the same volume or weight—than fresh fruit or vegetables. Studies have demonstrated an inverse association between the energy density of a diet and relative costs per unit of energy (Drewnowski & Darmon, 2005). Of course, there is considerable variation in terms of the cost of food depending on where it is bought and how highly processed it is—high-calorie fast food may remain more expensive, even on a per calorie basis, than healthier whole foods (McDermott & Stephens, 2010). However, when like is compared with like, healthier formulations tend to remain more costly (Temple et al., 2010). Undoing this disparity between the cost of food and its dietary effects may, therefore, be one way to address childhood obesity, at least if it can be shown that the cost of food affects food purchasing decisions.

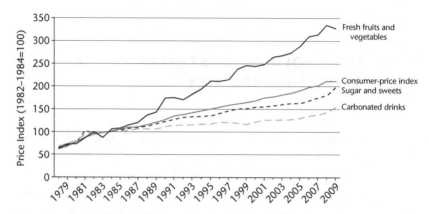

FIGURE 7.1 Relative Price Changes for Fresh Fruits and Vegetables, Sugars and Sweets, and Carbonated Drinks, 1978–2009

Source: Brownell and Frieden (2009, p. 1807); data are from the Bureau of Labor Statistics and represent the US city averages for all urban consumers in January of each year.

Yet policies to manipulate food prices raise important ethical and political issues. Where does responsibility lie for food purchases? Is there a role for government in food pricing structures? How would any new intervention fit with existing government measures that affect food production and pricing? Can such a policy be equitable? In this chapter we consider the potential for such policies, with particular attention to sugar-sweetened drinks (as a product consumed by many children that has attracted high-profile controversy) and effects on lower income families. We argue that the issues are too complex to permit knock-down arguments on either side. However, we do suggest that many objections to tax and subsidy measures as "nanny state" interference frame the issues much too simply. As we note at several points in this chapter, state action already affects absolute and relative food prices, often in ways that run counter to accepted nutritional advice. We therefore argue that this is an area where experimentation with different policies would be very welcome. In addition, we suggest that proposals for tax and subsidy policies are important just because they highlight how far existing food markets depart from the various hopes we invest in them—whether these concern free and fair competition, consumer choice, or children's health.

Background

Taxes on food are not a new idea. In the United States, taxes already exist in seventeen states and cover products such as syrups, candy, and fruit drinks (Mozaffarian et al., 2012). Likewise, in Canada a sales tax is applied to soft drinks, sweets, and snack foods, while other foods are free from sales tax. Food items are also differentially taxed across Europe—in the United Kingdom, for example, some food items such as confectionery, potato chips and savory snacks, and hot takeaways are subject to a sales tax (value added tax or VAT at 20 percent), while most foodstuffs are not (Caraher & Cowburn, 2007; Leicester & Windmeijer, 2004). These taxes clearly correspond to products considered to be less healthy, although their original rationale was often based in the undesirability of taxing the main food groups, viewed as essential items for every household.

In Denmark in 2011, as part of a wide-ranging tax reform, the government implemented a tax on food products such as meat, dairy products (except milk), animal fats, and vegetable oils. The tax applied where saturated fat content exceeded 2.3 percent, in proportion to the weight of saturated fats in the product (Nicholls et al., 2011a). Although the tax attracted considerable criticism—and has since been repealed[1]—other countries have followed suit (Villanueva, 2011). Hungary, for example, has introduced a tax on specific classes of food such as sweetened drinks, prepacked sweetened products, salty snacks, and condiments (Anonymous, 2011; Cain, 2011), while in France a tax on sweetened drinks has been introduced (Travers & Benoit-Guyod, 2012). The difference between existing taxes and these newer schemes lies principally in their rationale—recent proposals have the explicit aim of shifting purchasing patterns away from energy-dense, unhealthy foods toward more nutritious alternatives. It is perhaps worth adding, however, that there is a long history of tax policies oriented by public health concerns. For example, though less relevant to children, note that most governments specifically

---

1. In November 2012 the Danish tax ministry announced it would repeal the 2011 tax changes, including the levy on fats as well as a proposed (but not yet implemented) tax on sugar. A short-term study indicated a decrease in consumption of fats (butter, butter-blends, margarines, and oils) of 10–20 percent (Jensen & Smed, 2012), and that US$216 million was raised (Strom, 2012). However, the tax reportedly led to cross-border shopping to Sweden and Germany for goods affected by the new tax (Anonymous, 2012) and administrative difficulties for companies. As this suggests, the rationale for repealing the tax is an economic one, illustrating some of the complexities of policy making where—as we have stressed—health is not the only issue in play.

tax alcoholic drinks in order to discourage consumption (as well as to raise revenue).

Two further points about taxation policies and proposals are also worth making by way of introduction. First, note that such measures are politically more attractive if they are coupled with cross-subsidies. The revenues raised might be used to subsidize healthier foods or to fund prevention initiatives that target specific populations. For example, funds could be directed toward a measure like the European School Fruit Scheme. At present some member states, together with 90 million euro from European funds, provide finances that subsidize the cost of providing free fruit to school children (European Commission: Directorate-General for Agriculture and Rural Development, 2012). Whatever measures are chosen, the key point would be that the health-based rationale for such policies risks being diluted if they result in increases to general government revenue, since the tax then gives governments a stake in higher consumption levels of the taxed product. This effect can be countered if funds are specifically earmarked for activities that underline the original justification for the tax.[2]

Second, since new tax proposals naturally attract the charge of unwanted or unwarranted state interference, it is important to bear in mind how extensively governments already intervene in food markets. Sometimes this takes the form of active measures: subsidies, import taxes, support for agricultural research, spending on infrastructure, and regulatory measures. Many of these measures have led to decreases in retail food prices, although others actually increase costs to consumers. For example, in the United States the low prices of the common sweetener high-fructose corn syrup (and the sugared drinks that rely on it) are partly the result of subsidies and supports for corn. But the widespread adoption of this syrup by the American food industry has also been driven by the quotas and tariffs that the United States—contrary to all strictures about free trade—imposes on sugar imports, in order to support "US sugar prices above comparable levels in the world market" (United States Department of Agriculture Economic Research Service, 2012). Despite the formidable complexity of this and other subsidy schemes, most commentators agree that their net effect is to favor less healthy foodstuffs, and the processed food industry, by supporting the production of commodity crops and industrial meat, dairy, and poultry production (since these depend on soy and

---

2. Of course, if those activities are worthwhile, it might be argued that they should be funded from the fairest and most efficient forms of general taxation, rather than by a particular food-based tax (Strnad, 2004, p. 1226).

corn as feedstuffs). For example, one of the most important subsidies takes the form of government funding for agricultural research. This has focused on increased yield in meat and dairy products, storable commodities, and oilseeds, with much less funding devoted to fruits, vegetables, or forage crops (Muller et al., 2007).

In addition, there are important issues that arise from government *in*action. In many spheres of agriculture and food production there is a remarkable and culpable lack of government intervention. Some parts of the food supply chain effectively operate as cartels; others rely heavily on illegal labor practices; and many create sizeable negative externalities—costs to wider society that include pollution and health risks from new infectious agents and antibiotic resistance. By breaching their duty to ensure that markets function properly, governments play a hidden role in food pricing.[3] Sometimes the results favor producers over consumers; in many cases, the results also involve apparent benefits for consumers in the form of artificially cheap food. That is, food on supermarket shelves seems cheap, because its price does not reflect many of its actual costs, not to mention the future costs that are being accumulated by unsustainable food production systems (see further Guthman, 2011; Lawrence, 2008; Roberts, 2008). As we noted in chapter 6, these systemic problems are largely invisible. Consumption choices are a matter of everyday awareness, as is the fiercely competitive and diabolically clever marketing that promotes products high in "added value"—which in our context means highly processed foods and drinks. Unfortunately, the systems that set these prices and promote certain choices are much harder to appreciate and understand, making it more difficult to address important questions about power and alternatives.

Implementing a Fiscal Food Policy

Setting aside the complex background issues posed by subsidies, quotas, and regulation, there are two obvious ways in which governments can deliberately affect food prices. Particular foods might be taxed. Alternatively, some foods could be subsidized in order to make them (relatively) cheaper to consumers;

---

3. As discussed in chapter 3, one complexity in the relation between causation and responsibility is that persons and organizations can be (retrospectively) responsible for inaction, to the extent that they have (prospective) responsibilities to intervene.

or—perhaps more likely—other health-related facilities might be funded on the cross-subsidy model mentioned above. We now briefly review some current proposals for fiscal food policies (see also Cash & Lacanilao, 2007).

Point-of-Purchase Taxes

One possibility would be to adapt sales taxes in order to impose a simple percentage price levy at the point-of-purchase. Specific classes of food and drink could be increased in price, most likely on the basis of an assessment of whether they are "unhealthy"—for example, foods with high fat or sugar content. As already mentioned, several countries tax some foods in this way, whether because they are unhealthy or because they are deemed nonessential. Several studies of pricing effects, which we briefly discuss below, are based on such sales taxes as well. In theory, subsidies could also be applied in such a way, though we are not aware of any such proposals—more likely are selective measures, such as the School Fruit Scheme just mentioned, that target particular groups.

Depending on the ways in which foods are classified, a sales tax can also provide an incentive for manufacturers to reduce the amount of a taxed constituent within a product. This might either move the product out of the taxed category, or at least reduce the levy on it. Consequently, a sales tax might modify producer as well as consumer behavior and encourage the production of healthier food products. This approach has been successfully employed in several other contexts—for instance, to encourage the sale of unleaded car fuels (and the cars that use them) by taxing leaded fuel at a higher rate (Marshall, 2000).

An Excise Tax on Particular Constituents

An alternative approach is an excise tax, that is, a tax levied on a per unit basis, depending on constituents of the food or drink. The Danish tax on fat within foods is a form of excise tax. As in the previous case, this may encourage reformulating some products to bring them beneath this threshold. However, since the tax covers many unprocessed foods—such as butter and meats—this effect may not be significant. Some authors, such as Lustig et al. (2012), single out sugar as a particular target for taxation and liken it to alcohol in terms of its "unavoidability (or pervasiveness throughout society), toxicity, potential for abuse and negative impact on society" (p. 28). They therefore suggest taxing "processed foods that contain any form of added sugars.... This would include sweetened fizzy drinks (soda) and other sugar-sweetened beverages (for example, juice, sports drinks and chocolate milk), and also sugared cereal" (p. 29). This would have the benefit of targeting processed foods in particular, and of encouraging product reformulation to reduce overall sugar content. Rather differently, Okrent and Alston (2012) suggest that, economically speaking, the most efficient tax would be a tax based simply on the calorie content of foods.

An Excise Tax on Particular Food Groups

Some of the most prominent current proposals are more specific than either of these types of measures. They suggest that an excise tax be placed on particular foods such as snacks or sugar-sweetened drinks (Barry et al., 2009; Brownell & Frieden, 2009; Brownell et al., 2009; Cash & Lacanilao, 2007; Kuchler et al., 2004; Okrent & Alston, 2012).

The proposal most relevant to children's health is to impose a tax by volume on sugar-sweetened beverages—not just sodas, but also energy drinks, sweetened water, and fruit drinks—as advocated by Kelly Brownell et al. (Brownell et al., 2009; Friedman & Brownell, 2012). Proposals along these lines have been the subject of vigorous debate in the United States, particularly in New York where Governor David Patterson attempted to pass a one cent per fluid ounce soda tax in the annual budget of 2010—the second time he had done so (Wahba, 2010). However, New York is not the only place that has considered such a tax. Cities, including Richmond, California, are also balloting the voting public on such measures, while others such as Philadelphia have turned down tax proposals (Baertlein & Geller, 2012). In the United Kingdom, a soda tax is reportedly being considered by the Liberal Democrats (Bailey, 2012), while the Academy of Medical Royal Colleges (2013) has called for a tax of at least 20 percent on sugary drinks for a one-year trial period.

Such proposals naturally invite the charge of arbitrariness in singling out just one class of products when—as the food industry invariably points out—overall consumption of many different products (not to mention low levels of physical activity) may be the over-arching causal factors. Advocates of taxes on sugar-sweetened drinks have important arguments on their side, however. In the United States, soda consumption has risen five-fold over the last three decades and now provides about seven percent of calories in the average diet (Claro et al., 2012). In children, consumption of sweetened drinks may account for 10–15 percent of calories consumed (Brownell & Frieden, 2009).

These calories are in the form of simple sugars: repeated encounters with this high glycemic load increase the risk of diabetes and cardiovascular problems (Ludwig, 2002), not to mention damage to tooth enamel. Moreover, the drinks contain no other nutrients of value: there is actually no reason why any child should ever drink them. Not least, there is evidence that soft drinks bypass normal satiety signals (Vartanian et al., 2007), which explains how some children—and adults—are capable of consuming such large quantities. Of all the products regularly consumed by children, sugar-sweetened drinks have a special claim on our attention.

An excise tax—whether on the volume of a sweetened drink or on the content a particular constituent such as sugar—has a notable advantage over seemingly more straightforward point-of-purchase sales taxes. This is because it can be structured to avoid "bulk buying" incentives. On a normal sales tax, a large soda would be taxed at the same percentage rate as a small one. This is problematic because, like many of the foods often implicated in childhood obesity, sodas have been subject to the well-known marketing strategy of "supersizing"—that is, offering greater perceived value by selling larger servings or packs at much lower costs per volume or weight. A sales tax based simply on purchase price therefore favors larger quantities. A levy based on volume or the amount of a particular nutrient content avoids this since the tax would increase proportionately with volume or weight.

Limits on Quantities Sold

Although it is neither a tax nor a subsidy, the recent proposal—subject to legal wrangling in New York as we write—to limit the volumes of soft drinks sold has important price implications. The New York measure limits sales of sweetened drinks in restaurants (and some other venues) to servings of 16 ounces or half a liter—to European eyes already a rather large serving. The effect is to raise the price per volume, because it blocks the common retail strategy (just mentioned) of reducing prices of larger volumes in order to enhance perceived value and increase turnover. Where serving sizes are limited, someone who wants a "Big Gulp"—32 ounces—must buy two of the largest size drinks on offer and hence pay twice as much. (Evidently, the same maths applies twice over to a 64-ounce "Double Big Gulp.") The soda proposal is probably a special case, however. Despite the popularity of "supersizing" among fast-food chains and the growth of portion sizes in most US restaurants, it is obviously difficult to legislate for maximum portion sizes in the case of foods, or to devise other legal strategies to discourage the sale of oversized portions.

Modification of Existing Subsidies

As briefly discussed above, governments already intervene extensively in food prices. A further option would therefore be to modify existing fiscal measures, such as the agricultural subsidies provided as part of the European Common Agricultural Policy or the US Farm Bill. As mentioned, subsidies tend to support the production of less healthy food items, especially storable commodities such as wheat, soy, corn, and even sugar and hence to support the poultry and meat industries, which rely on cheap feedstuffs. Insofar as subsidies decrease food costs, it is argued that this leads to increased purchasing and hence higher levels of obesity (Elinder, 2005; Lang & Rayner, 2005).

However, subsidy schemes are invariably complex in structure and involve many regulatory provisions; and they often have indirect effects, such as driving up the price of agricultural land. Indeed, some subsidy schemes are designed to support prices to farmers and hence increase prices to consumers. For example, one of the few subsidy schemes for fruits and vegetables is the European Union's "withdrawal support" scheme: "When the price drops below a specified intervention level, the EU finances the withdrawal of fruits and vegetables from the market.... Most of this surplus is destroyed. In other words, the EU policy keeps prices high by limiting availability" (Veerman et al., 2006, p. 31). Because of such complexities, altering subsidies to farmers and agribusinesses may not have the expected effect on consumer food prices (Alston et al., 2008; Miller & Coble, 2007; Mozaffarian et al., 2012). More generally, as Barry Popkin (2011) observes, "a huge disconnect exists between the prices farmers receive for a product and its retail cost. For instance, the prices that farmers receive for fruits and vegetables have declined in real terms during the past 40 years, but the prices that consumers pay have increased. In other words, farmers are not receiving the extra money—this goes to the middlemen, agribusinesses and major food chains" (p. 16).

Consequently, although there are good arguments to alter many existing incentive and subsidy schemes, more immediate effects can be expected from direct measures such as excise or sales taxes. Although it goes beyond our scope here, it is also worth noting that more direct effects might be achieved by addressing aspects of the supply chain, such as indirect subsidies and regulatory failures. For example, shifting government support toward more local food distribution structures, challenging anticompetitive business practices, or regulating safety hazards (such as the use of antibiotics to promote rapid growth of livestock) could all redress some of the unhelpful shifts in the relative prices of different foodstuffs that we mentioned at the beginning of this chapter.

Food Costs, Purchases, and Health

Of course, the relevance of tax measures depends on there being an association between the price of food, purchasing patterns, and, ultimately, people's health. A number of studies now support this association and indicate that price is a key component in food purchasing decisions, particularly for lower income families (Mhurchu et al., 2010; Mozaffarian et al., 2012; Waterlander et al., 2010). Some authors also observe that consumer perceptions may not correspond to actual availability and price, and that such perceptions have additional effects. Since food companies spend considerable resources persuading us that their products represent good value—especially those products with the greatest "added value"—we should be wary of assuming that consumer perceptions correspond to the actualities. (See Giskes et al. [2007] for references, as well as a cautious view of these effects.)

Price manipulation studies show that price reductions of healthier foods increase sales. This has been demonstrated in the context of vending machine sales (French et al., 2001), school canteens, and controlled laboratory studies of supermarket expenditure (Epstein et al., 2007; Epstein et al., 2010). Using data from a nationally representative sample of US adolescents Powell et al. (2009) found that fruit and vegetable consumption was significantly associated with price, with a $1 increase in price being associated with a reduction in weekly consumption by almost one-third. Equally, a point-of-purchase intervention study within a hospital setting found that sales of soft drinks decreased in line with the imposed price increase (Block et al., 2010). In several experiments involving price manipulations within a supermarket environment, Ni Mhurchu et al. (2010, 2007) found that an increase in price results in a decrease in the sales of these items. These findings suggest that policies which manipulate price structures through the taxation of unhealthy foods and subsidization of healthy foods may be a useful tool in reducing levels of childhood obesity, at least insofar as these policies are widely recognized by consumers.

Despite this evidence, some authors suggest that price manipulation policies are likely to be ineffective. Oliver (2006), for instance, contends that "if you wanted to reduce soda consumption by half, you would have to make a can of coke cost about four dollars" (p. 174). However, we believe such pessimism is overstated and reflects a misleading hope for a simple, single solution—a silver bullet—to address "the issue." As we argued in chapter 2, the important question is not whether an initiative or policy will, on its own, make a decisive difference to childhood obesity rates or related health problems. As Brownell et al. (2009) observe, "Seat-belt legislation and tobacco taxation do not eliminate traffic accidents and heart disease but are nevertheless sound policies" (p. 1603). In other words, we need to consider whether a measure can make a helpful contribution, at the same time as being congruent with other goals of public policy. Even small changes in diet at the population level—far less than the 50 percent reduction in soda consumption that Oliver mentions—are likely to have beneficial effects.

The Ethics of Taxation

However, effectiveness is not the only issue. Tax and subsidy policies are political measures that enact powerful collective judgments. As one journalist nicely put it:

> what soda tax opponents don't want to admit is that a levy on sugared water can be an effective weapon in that it represents a powerful message. It puts soda squarely in the cigarette and alcohol category as something that we as a society need to either cut back on or stomp out, or at least tax in order to fund programs that will counter the horrible effects. (M. Warner, 2010)

In other words, such policies are not only to be judged by their immediate effects, but also by the moral and political claims that they make. This is something that their opponents will readily agree on—except that they view those claims quite differently. Even if it could be shown that tax and subsidy policies would make a significant contribution to obesity levels or overall health, opponents tend to interpret such measures as resting on overbearing claims about state authority. In slightly different terms, there are important questions as to whether tax and subsidy policies can cohere with the other responsibilities of government, and whether they may complement or disrupt the proper responsibilities of companies, parents, and individuals.

In the following sections, we will focus on two main normative arguments against such policies: that taxation is paternalistic, and that taxation would be regressive—that is, would disproportionately affect those on lower incomes. Against the charge of paternalism, we will raise several points that suggest the issue is not so simple. Measures that enjoy wide public support are not aptly described as paternalistic, at least in any pejorative sense; and much depends, we believe, on the appropriate framing of the issues. We will also argue that concerns about the possible regressive effects of tax measures can be addressed by coupling taxes with subsidies for healthier foods or other measures that promote healthier diets, and by carefully considering (both in design and in evaluation) their overall effects on the health and welfare of different groups.

Taxation and Subsidy Is Paternalistic

Advocates of tax and subsidy measures typically invoke a justification in terms of public health. Critics may respond that this unreasonably expands the scope of public health, from the containment of contagious diseases (which few would disagree is an important government responsibility) to the reduction or prevention of nontransmissible conditions such as obesity (e.g., Epstein, 2003). In other words, "public health" is being invoked to justify measures that—as critics would have it—protect people from themselves. Put this way, the question of paternalism[4] is unavoidable: "prohibitions or sanctions on the purchase or sale of problematic foods… constitute paternalism in the private sphere, at odds with mainstream conceptions of liberty in democratic societies" (Bloche, 2004).

Note first, however, that tax and subsidy schemes may be motivated by concerns other than individuals' health. Many commentators focus on increased health care costs, which are passed on to taxpayers wherever such costs are supported by taxation (e.g., Marshall, 2000). Focusing on policies' potential to reduce costs to others, or to meet costs that would otherwise be imposed on others, allows proponents to avoid the charge of paternalism. This line of argument has been pursued, for example, in connection with motorcycle helmet laws (Jones & Bayer, 2007) and smoking (Bayer & Colgrove, 2002). While this may be "the main argument for public intervention from a strictly economic perspective" (Jensen & Smed, 2007, p. 2), however, it is still problematic. This is partly because the exact associations between particular health conditions and the costs they create are highly contentious, for reasons we mentioned in chapter 1. A purely economic rationale is also problematic for the moral and political reasons that we considered in chapter 2: it views costs of treatment as unwanted burdens rather than help offered in a spirit of solidarity.

---

4. As noted in chapter 6, claims about paternalism need to be framed somewhat differently when it is children's health that is the focus of our attention—a point we set aside here. For definitions and detailed discussion of paternalism, see Nys (2008) and Dworkin (2010).

A more promising response, we believe, is to follow Gerald Dworkin (2010) and Peter de Marneffe (2006), who suggest that "paternalism" is not intrinsically problematic. As Jones and Bayer (2007) argue with respect to motorcycle helmet legislation, the "challenge for public health is to expand on [the] base of *justified* paternalism" (p. 216). We can conceptualize the problem of paternalism as involving the conflict between two duties: the duty to promote the well-being of others and the duty to respect their choices (Archard, 1990). While it is contentious to ascribe to the state a generalized duty to promote well-being, it is much less controversial to say that it should take the effects on people's well-being into account as it pursues other activities. Thus, rather than allow the charge of paternalism to become a "conversation stopper," we should consider how these two duties—to protect both individuals' health and well-being and their liberty or autonomy—are enacted in particular policies.

The first point to note is that taxation involves a relatively minor restriction on individual liberty, compared with outright bans or laws proscribing certain behaviors. It does not remove choice, but alters the balance of costs and opportunities—it makes healthy choices easier and unhealthy choices more costly. Moreover, current proposals to tax particular foods are far from the levels that have been imposed on products such as tobacco, which in some countries amount to over 75 percent of the purchase price (Mackay & Eriksen, 2002). The levels of taxation being proposed are dissuasive rather than restrictive or prohibitive.

More than this, there is not a simple trade-off between welfare and liberty here. In some instances, restrictions on individual liberty can *enhance* individual autonomy—for example when policies interfere with activities that could threaten individuals' physical or mental health or their ability to think for themselves, or that might leave them dependent on others (de Marneffe, 2006, p. 81). Analogously, schemes that combine taxes and subsidies may actually *enhance* individuals' effective spheres of choice, if they address some of the structural barriers that prevent individuals from adopting healthy behaviors (see also Buchanan, 2008). On this argument, tax-subsidy schemes, while restricting liberty to some extent, could also be autonomy-promoting as they enhance individuals' and families' abilities to adopt a healthier diet.

Furthermore, when people consent to have their liberties restricted, such restrictions cease to be paternalistic. After all, what we want to do in the moment does not always reflect our more considered judgment. As we highlighted in chapter 6, markets airbrush out many difficult background realities. So we may easily be tempted to buy products such as clothes produced in sweatshops, or fruits picked by exploited migrant workers. On reflection or debate, however, it is possible to step back and consider the systems and practices behind the choices that companies are offering us. Taking this broader perspective may well lead us to judge that some choices should never have been available in the first place. Policies that broadly cohere with public attitudes and enjoy a democratic mandate are certainly less paternalistic than those that do not. It should be added that where policies are likely to affect some people more than others—for example, parents on lower incomes— there will be a special argument for ensuring that those voices and interests are heeded in the political process. In any event, where that process operates democratically, we may exercise our freedom as citizens in order to limit or alter the choices that are open to us as consumers (G. Williams, 2012a; see O'Neill, 2002, p. 169ff for a more skeptical view).

Public Attitudes to Taxation and Subsidization

This brings us directly to the question of public attitudes and debate. Historically, there has been considerable resistance to the imposition of taxes on food items. As an anonymous discussion in the *Harvard Law Review* (2003) points out:

> A significant factor in evaluating the political practicability of state paternalism is the extent to which government action infringes individual autonomy relative to the perceived benefits of the intervention. This factor does not call for rough quantitative balancing, but rather assesses the degree to which the activity in question is associated with the individual's identity. So, for example, mandatory seat belt and motorcycle helmet laws, though clearly on the strong end of the paternalism spectrum, have gained general acceptance because the costs they impose on autonomy are minor relative to the benefits they confer in safety…paternalism in this instance is not truly offensive…because few people would consider their decision to forego the use of seat belts an expression of their true selves. (p. 1174)

As the same author points out, dietary habits—and, one might add, parenting behavior—are very much bound up with individuals' identities, which is one reason why debates in these areas are often extremely heated.

However, recent survey data suggest that public attitudes may be thawing, and several studies report increasing support for tax-based interventions

(Oliver & Lee, 2005; Rudd Center for Food Policy & Obesity, 2009). A 2003 Health Pulse of America survey found that 27 percent of those surveyed were in favor of a government tax on snack foods as an effort to reduce obesity. When the same question was posed as part of the Harvard School of Public Health Obesity Survey, 41 percent were in favor. In the United Kingdom, a 2010 survey of university students found that 51.9 percent supported a raise in taxes on the sale of unhealthy foods (Okonkwo & While, 2010). As we indicated, particularly relevant are the opinions of those likely to be affected the most, in this case lower income families. Our own research with European families suggested that while support for policies of taxation and subsidy was relatively high, it was actually greater among low-income parents (Nicholls et al., 2011b; but compare Suggs & McIntyre, 2011). In focus group research conducted in deprived neighborhoods in the Netherlands, the option of increasing the costs of unhealthy foods and reducing the costs of healthy foods was spontaneously offered by participants (Waterlander et al., 2010). This suggests that far from being paternalistic, a price manipulation policy may be welcomed by those affected, including—and perhaps especially—low-income families.

An inevitable limitation of such research is that responses vary considerably depending on the framing of the question and details of the proposal. For example, responses are clearly affected by the inclusion of specific details about how taxes and subsidies may be used. In a 2008 survey conducted for the Citizens Committee for Children of New York, parents were asked:

> Some leaders in New York state are considering charging a one cent tax per ounce on all sugar-sweetened beverages—such as soda and sports drinks—and using a portion of the money to combat obesity in children and adults. Sugar-sweetened beverages do not include diet soda or seltzer. Based on what you know, would you support or oppose this new tax?

Over half (52 percent) of respondents supported such a tax to some degree with one-third (33 percent) strongly supporting the measure. In a further question, participants were asked:

> Supporters of a penny-per-ounce tax on sugar-sweetened beverages say it will raise up to $1 billion to help fund effective programs to combat obesity in children and adults. It will also help close the state budget deficit of $14 billion, reducing the need to raise property taxes and

sales taxes or impose massive cuts on schools, health care, mass transit, or law enforcement. Based on what you just learned, would you support or oppose this new tax?

This elicited an increase in support with 72 percent of respondents now supporting the measure to some degree and half strongly supporting it (Beck Research Inc., LLC, 2008). The much stronger wording (the funding of effective programs), together with explicit financial information (amounts rather than percentages; undertakings not to raise taxes in other areas), appear to affect attitudes considerably.

Of course, it is no surprise that support depends both on how questions are framed and specific aspects of the policy proposed. Political debates invariably concern different ways of framing the issue. In large part, disagreements about the ethics of taxation reflect different ways of understanding current policies and possible interventions. We have already hinted at one way in which we think it is helpful to frame—or rather reframe—the issues. When opponents of tax-subsidy measures, or other government interventions, argue that such policies would distort markets, restrict legitimate commercial interests, or limit consumer freedom, they invoke ideals of free markets and consumer choice. However valid those ideals, the fact is that modern food systems are not free markets, and they do not simply reflect consumer demand. As mentioned already in this chapter, all sorts of factors—including government intervention in food production and failures of competition—affect food pricing and availability. A small number of very large companies invest heavily to modify and shape consumer preferences, in line with their own interest in "adding value"—that is, selling heavily processed and easily consumed foods based on the cheapest and most widely available ingredients. The results do not correspond to an economic or political ideal of free markets, any more than they are ideal from a health point of view. In other words, while tax-subsidy proposals are often rejected as misplaced attempts to protect people from their own choices, one might equally interpret them as ways to protect consumers from a series of factors that distort food marketing, availability, and prices.

Nonetheless, it might be felt that there is something perverse about imposing fiscal measures to support healthy diets, so as to counteract a raft of subsidies, regulations, and policies that encourage the availability of less healthy foods. If governments have proved irrational or if their agencies have often been captured by vested interests, why should we think they will do better with fiscal interventions? Much simpler, it might be said, to undo the originally problematic measures or to remedy current failures in regulation and competition. Although achieving those things in practice would be far from simple, we would not disagree with the overall line of thought. Rather, we consider it a virtue of this way of framing matters that these broader structural or (in the terms of the previous chapter) environmental issues are raised for scrutiny. For this reason, we will conclude this chapter by suggesting that it may make sense to view tax and subsidy proposals not so much as solutions, but instead in two rather different ways: as helpful experiments and as provocations that encourage us to face larger problems of modern food systems.

For the moment, however, our main point is that the charge of paternalism should not be seen as a decisive argument against fiscal policies that aim to change consumption patterns. Such schemes involve relatively minor restrictions on individual liberty; they have the potential to enhance parents' ability to feed their children healthily; and—depending on how they are debated, justified, and designed—they may meet with widespread public approval.

Taxation Policies Would Be Regressive

A second common argument against proposed taxation policies is that they would be regressive—that is, those on lower incomes are likely to pay a greater proportion of their income on the tax. This argument can be made irrespective of the form of tax, since in each case the end result is likely to be that costs are passed on to consumers, and food represents a larger proportion of expenditure in poorer households (Cash & Lacanilao, 2007; P. Williams et al., 2007). It is already clear that price serves as a significant barrier when purchasing a healthy diet, above all for poorer families (Inglis et al., 2005; Slater et al., 2009; Waterlander et al., 2010; P. Williams et al., 2007).

In large part, this is an empirical question that must remain open until there is greater experience of such policies. As Jensen and Smed (2007) note, "empirical experience with regard to differentiated food taxes—and thus empirical evidence about the effects of food taxation on food consumption and health—is practically non-existing" (p. 2). In the meantime, attempts to model the impacts of policies depend on many assumptions and are open to many uncertainties.

In simulation studies, Nnoaham et al. (2009) found that a policy of taxation accompanied by a price reduction of 17.5 percent on fruits and vegetables would not only improve food purchasing, it would also generate over £10 billion and decrease annual deaths from coronary heart disease, stroke, and cancer, with a greater effect in lower income families. In an international comparison of different interventions, measures to increase the cost of unhealthy foods and decrease those of healthy foods were consistently predicted to be cost-saving in all the low-income and middle-income countries included, second only to advertising regulation in terms of the beneficial health effects generated in long-term models (Cecchini et al., 2010). Furthermore, in each country evaluated, the use of fiscal measures represented a cost saving after both 20 and 50 years with a sum of almost 500,000 Disability Adjusted Life Years (DALYs) averted every year. Other analyses also suggest that a taxation policy would be both effective and cost-effective (Sacks et al., 2011).

However, as Schroeter et al. (2008) have argued, while the law of demand suggests that there is an inverse relationship between the price of a good and the quantity of the good consumed, "it is not necessarily the case that [average body] weight will also decline when ready substitutes are available" (p. 47). For example, one modeling scenario indicated that while a tax on foods high in saturated fats could reduce saturated fat consumption, it also tended to increase salt consumption. Furthermore, fruit consumption tended to fall as a result of taxation on milk and cream (Mytton et al., 2007). These results indicate how the highly interdependent nature of food consumption makes effects difficult to predict. An earlier experience in Denmark also provides empirical evidence for these complexities. Following the implementation of a 1976 tax on sugar, there was both a period of consumer hoarding but also a move from traditional sugar products to alternative sugars made from nontaxed ingredients such as maize starch (Danish Academy of Technical Sciences, 2007). Many further uncertainties attend attempts to model such impacts.

At the same time, as we discussed in chapter 2, complexity and uncertainty are not arguments for inaction, and other possible benefits need to be borne in mind. Policies addressing the price of food may have benefits that are not immediately apparent. Consider the effect that redesigned farm subsidies could have, for example. Subsidy schemes could be altered to favor fruits and vegetables (as opposed to commodity crops), to support smaller growers (unlike most existing agricultural subsidies), to promote local food distribution (as opposed to the distribution networks of a few transnational commodity companies), to enhance crop diversity (as opposed to increasingly risky and unsustainable monocultures), and so on. As we have been urging throughout this book, policy-making should be informed by many ends. One of the key problems with modern food systems is that so much agricultural policy has been badly distorted by an over-emphasis on commodity production, not to mention vested interests that have gained a hold through decades of lobbying and pork-barrel politics and a wider lack of transparency and public scrutiny.

There is also a more specific question about whether food taxes—if they do have regressive effects—should be considered unjust, especially if it is possible to channel their benefits toward poorer individuals and families. In the context of tobacco taxation, for example, it has been suggested that those on lower incomes are more sensitive to price and therefore more likely than more affluent smokers to change their behavior in response to increases to taxation (Siahpush et al., 2009; Wilson & Thomson, 2005). A similar argument could be made in the context of food pricing. US data for children and young adults has suggested that those from the lowest income group are most sensitive to the price of fruits and vegetables (Powell & Chaloupka, 2009; Sturm & Datar, 2010). In the context of unhealthy food, it should also be borne in mind that "obesity and diabetes are regressive diseases that affect the poor in greater numbers" (Brownell et al., 2010). For this reason, lower income groups have more to gain from the taxation of unhealthy products, making taxation policies "a 'progressive' public health policy" (Warner, 2000, p. 84). Depending on their exact design, tax-subsidy policies may help address one of the structural barriers that low-SES groups face in adopting healthy diets. As such, there may be an argument from justice for a fiscal food policy.

Of course, as we have argued throughout, we should not expect a single policy option to provide a wholesale solution to childhood obesity, never mind broader health inequalities. Price is only one barrier to healthy food purchasing; personal, institutional, informational, and infrastructural barriers remain for low-income families (Nicholls et al., 2011a). Only approaches that tackle diverse policy domains are likely to address childhood obesity and reduce existing health inequalities on a long-term basis. Still, policies of taxation and subsidy may make a valuable contribution to addressing the obesogenic environment, reducing health inequalities, and enabling lower income groups to buy healthier foods.

Conclusion

In this chapter we have discussed one key aspect of our obesogenic environment: how food and drink prices work as a specific driver of unhealthy consumption patterns and increasing rates of childhood obesity. We have also countered some common objections to deliberate interference in food prices. Against the charge that such policies would be paternalistic, we have argued that these policies need not be heavily restrictive and may in fact be autonomy-promoting for families who currently can least afford a healthy diet. We have also pointed to evidence of increasing public support for these policies. Against the charge that such taxes would be regressive and unfair to poorer families, we have pointed out that such policies may generate greater benefits for lower income families. Much will depend on the design of such measures and how the revenue gained is deployed, however, and the views of less well-off parents deserve special consideration.

Of course, any such scheme will have to answer many practical questions, such as the level of taxation, the foods affected, and the ways in which subsidies are applied or the funds raised are used. While these issues are complex and important, they do not involve in-principle objections to such policies. Rather, they suggest that there are many questions of judgment and implementation that are unlikely to be addressed even by the most thorough advance discussions. In other words, we should see this as an area that is ripe for political experimentation and policy learning. We therefore conclude this chapter with two somewhat different thoughts, which reflect our ambivalence about the various tax proposals that are currently being debated and enacted.

In the first place, we would like to suggest that new fiscal policies should be taken as valuable *experiments* (see Academy of Medical Royal Colleges, 2013). It is clear that enough dissatisfaction has built up with current structures of food and drink markets that some such policies will be implemented, both in Europe and in some American states. These examples will rightly attract considerable scrutiny, as has the short-lived Danish experience. They can be looked at as experiments in public policy that offer unique opportunities to study effects on consumer behavior and consumption patterns, on different socioeconomic groups, and on people's health, including both children's and adults' obesity rates.

Second, we believe that tax-subsidy proposals should be taken as important *provocations*. Even if one disagrees that fiscal measures would be wise or effective, these proposals pose a vital question: How far do food markets and current modes of state intervention in them really serve people's interests? Increasing rates of childhood, and adult, obesity are just one reason for dissatisfaction. Behind a carefully marketed surface of plenty and convenience, of "choice" and "value," lies a whole set of problems in the workings of our food systems that we have only gestured at in this and the previous chapter. To cite a phrase we have used before, "Something Must Be Done." But given the formidable complexity of modern food systems and governments' interventions in them, the nature of that "something" is extremely difficult to judge. To reach considered judgments above sensible reforms one would have to take many other priorities into account—not least, enormous and urgent issues of sustainability and food security that go much beyond the scope of this book. In the meantime, tax and subsidy proposals pose a crucial question: If they are not "the" answer—and as we argue throughout this book, there is never one answer to complex policy questions—then what should be done to help make sure that our food systems address children's health and well-being, as well as the many other demands that they must serve?

RESPONDING TO FOOD MARKETING TARGETED AT CHILDREN

REGULATION, SOCIAL MARKETING, AND MEDIA LITERACY

Advertising targeted at children, much of which promotes foods high in salt, sugar, and fat, is often named as a central feature of the obesogenic environment and as a key contributing factor to the rise in childhood obesity. In this chapter, we summarize some of the available evidence on the effects of such advertising to children and consider three possible policy responses. First, some countries, such as Sweden and the United Kingdom, have implemented partial bans on advertising that targets children. Second, social marketers draw upon the tools and methods of commercial marketing to develop initiatives that promote physical activity and healthy nutrition among children. Third, media literacy education focuses on enabling children to decode marketing messages and may therefore make them less susceptible to marketing for unhealthy foods. We outline possible ways in which each of these strategies could be implemented to tackle childhood obesity and consider the strengths and limitations of each approach. As with many other anti-obesity measures, there is not sufficient evidence to prove that any one of these strategies on its own could make substantial contributions to ensuring healthier diets among children. Nonetheless, these strategies may complement one another and could be important planks in a broader strategy to address childhood obesity.

Marketing is a wider category than advertising and it might be argued that is it not enough to discuss advertising alone. As one author puts it, "When children see advertising that is aimed at them, invariably it has been aimed at them because marketers have developed a product or service with a high probability of being agreeable to children. When that advertising is successful in generating demand, it is therefore not surprising" (Preston, 2004, p. 368). In other words, heated as debates about advertising to children have been, the background to them is often taken for granted. For at least a century, food and drink companies have been aware of children as a distinct market and have formulated products specifically aimed at them. Sophisticated techniques of product formulation, testing, manufacture, and packaging (Kessler, 2009) stand behind the more obvious marketing strategies designed to promote these wares. These systems represent a structural feature of modern economies—it is highly unlikely, for example, that food and drink companies might cease to formulate products that target children's particular tastes. Likewise, it is hard to imagine regulatory measures that would rule out such products.[1]

In this chapter, then, we largely accept this situation as the environment in which parents and policy makers must act and focus on the narrower issue of advertising that aims to increase children's consumption of the various highly processed, attractively packaged, hyperpalatable foods and drinks that are being designed for them. As we noted in chapter 3, food manufacturers may claim, with some truth, that their individual products are safe for consumption. But those companies cannot honestly deny that they have material interests in encouraging the largest possible sales of such artificial foodstuffs and basing them on the cheapest ingredients available. And children manifestly need to be protected from excess consumption of them.

In this situation, parents find themselves caught in the middle, with the unenviable responsibility of protecting children from their easily stimulated desires for "kids' food."[2] Particularly invidious, in our view, are the ways in which companies have exploited strategies to bypass parents—for instance, by placing vending machines in schools or distributing educational materials that contain commercial messages. Lobstein (2009) gives the example of "counting books which use branded confectionery…to teach children numbers" (p. 882). More widely, the sheer "inequality of arms" between children and advertisers is deeply problematic: it enables commercial forces to enter into

---

1. This said, measures to encourage product reformulation (for instance, to reduce the amount of salt and sugar in breakfast cereals) are possible. Some fiscal measures mentioned in the last chapter might have this effect, as might food labeling requirements—for example, traffic light labeling involves marking a product as red, amber, or green in terms of key aspects of nutrient composition. This gives companies a clear incentive to make sure that their products fall on the green or amber side of the relevant thresholds. For another perspective—that the basic issue concerns overconsumption of processed foods, something that is naturally unaffected by product reformulation—see Monteiro (2009, 2010), as well as Michael Pollan's (2008) critique of "edible food-like substances."

2. As we discuss in chapter 9, this responsibility extends to those who act *in loco parentis*, that is, schools. For a recent US survey of parents' own views, see Harris et al. (2012).

family dynamics, affecting parents' authority to determine their children's food choices. As we argue in this chapter, even if we accept the production of "kids' foods" as part of modern food systems, these problems justify both pressure and regulation on companies to moderate their efforts to target children.

Children and Advertising

Many studies confirm that children are exposed to advertising from a variety of sources, much of it for highly palatable foods and drinks that have little nutritional value. Perhaps most significant in this area is the systematic review by Hastings et al. (2006). This has since been updated to take account of developments in both high- and low-income countries (Cairns et al., 2009).

Food is prominent among the products advertised to children. Hastings et al. (2004) find that "food is promoted to children more than any other product, apart from toys (and then only at Christmas)" (p. 19). Other researchers have found a similar emphasis on food, beverages, and fast-food restaurants in television advertising targeted at children (Brand, 2007; Powell et al., 2007). Foods high in fat, salt, and sugar are far more prevalent in advertisements targeting children than foods that meet core dietary requirements. Similarly, Hastings et al. find that television advertising promotes sugared breakfast cereals, soft drinks, sweet and savory snacks as well as fast-food brands. As they emphasize, the diet advertised to children stands in marked contrast with recommended guidelines on healthy nutrition (Hastings et al., 2006; Jones et al., 2006). TV advertising is generally the most frequently used medium (Hastings et al., 2004; Hastings et al., 2009; Matthews, 2008; Stead et al., 2007), with advertisers focusing on time slots relevant for children, such as weekend mornings or after-school hours during the week (Hastings et al., 2006). Children's exposure to TV advertising varies across countries. In the United States, recent estimates suggest that children see 11.5 minutes of such advertising per day (Goris et al., 2010). Figures appear to be lower in Europe: the same authors estimate exposure in Italy, Sweden, the United Kingdom, and the Netherlands at 6.2, 2.9, 2.4, and 1.8 minutes per day, respectively. Product placement in television shows and films also represents a less easily measured form of exposure (Skatrud-Mickelson et al., 2012; Speers et al., 2011; Sutherland et al., 2010). In addition, other media appear to be gaining momentum, such as the Internet (Cheyne et al., 2013), print media, or free gifts with food items and are beginning to be studied in more detail. Some researchers suggest that the importance of TV advertising may have begun to diminish, particularly in light of the rise of digital media (Cairns et al., 2009).

Whichever medium we are looking at, marketers are using carefully honed and highly effective persuasive techniques in their efforts to reach children (Kelly et al., 2010). This includes the use of fantasy themes, promotional techniques such as free gifts and toys, celebrities, and cartoon characters (Cairns et al., 2009; Hastings et al., 2006; Jones et al., 2006; Stead et al., 2007). Emotional appeals—linking products to fun, happiness, play, and peer acceptance, for example, are also employed (Page & Brewster, 2007).

How do these marketing efforts affect children? Different methods are used to determine the impact of food advertising on children. Some studies consider the relationships between exposure to advertisements and levels of obesity. Lobstein and Dibb (2005), for example, examine the link between advertising to children and the risk of overweight. They find a positive association—which may or may not indicate a causal connection—between the proportion of children overweight and the numbers of advertisements per hour on children's television, on the basis of data from the United States, Australia, and eight European countries.

Other studies try to assess the effects of marketing exposure on children directly to give a better sense of possible causal relations. Based on their review of the literature, Hastings et al. (2006) identify many different types of effects: "recall of food advertising, liking for and attitudes towards food advertising, communication about food advertising, purchase-request behaviour perceived to be triggered by food promotion, responses to free gifts and packaging, food preferences, food purchase behaviour, and food consumption behaviour" (p. 25; see further Epstein et al., 2008; Harris et al., 2009a, 2009c). In a different report, they conclude that

> evidence from many of the more complex studies, capable of inferring causality, demonstrate a statistically significant association between food promotion and children's knowledge, attitudes, behaviors and health status.... There is...evidence that food promotion influences children's food preferences, and encourages purchase and purchase requests to parents for the advertised foods. Food promotion was also found to influence children's consumption and other diet-related outcomes. These effects are significant, independent of other influences and operate at both brand and category level [that is, children come

to prefer both particular brands advertised, and the *categories* of foods that are advertised]. (Cairns et al., 2009, p. 32)

A further question concerns how children's cognitive development affects their ability to recognize marketing and how this might mediate the influence of (particular types of) advertising. It is not clear, for example, whether younger children—who have less understanding of the persuasive intent of advertising than older children—are more or less susceptible to advertising than older children. Brand (2007) points to two "critical stages" in children's ability to understand important features of television advertising. At five or six years of age, most children begin to be able to distinguish advertising from program content. At around age seven, they begin to recognize advertising as such. Children between the ages of two and six therefore "tend to view commercials as a form of on-going entertainment in line with programs they are watching" (p. 20; see also Moore, 2004).

More recently, it has been suggested that even if children recognize the selling intent of particular advertisements at around this age—that is, they appreciate that the advertiser is presenting information in order that viewers will buy the product—it may be a further and more important question whether they recognize the *persuasive* intent of advertising. As defined by Roberts (1983), this requires an appreciation

(1) that the source has other perspectives, hence other interests, than those of the receiver; (2) that the source intends to persuade; (3) that persuasive messages are, by definition, biased; (4) that biased messages demand different interpretation strategies than do primarily informational (or educational or entertainment) messages. (p. 27)

That is, children must understand that advertisers are not just presenting information about their product; they are using particular techniques to make the product more appealing and "attempting to make viewers do something they might not otherwise do" (Carter et al., 2011, p. 963). The ability to recognize persuasive as opposed to selling intent may not develop until much later, around 12 years of age (Carter et al., 2011).

Children's limited ability to recognize the purposes of advertising raises obvious ethical concerns. In particular, if children do not understand that advertisers' interests are distinct from, and may run counter to, their own, then their stance toward advertisements is one of unwarranted trust and vulnerability. However, it should also be noted that the greater cognitive skills of older children may make them *more* receptive to advertising:

> The fact that older children are both more attentive to entertainment in advertising, and better able to integrate what they are exposed to across multiple media suggests that continuing concern is warranted for this age group. Equipped with the ability to integrate the fantasy in the ad with the brand reality, yet not ready to enlist their defenses spontaneously, these children may be particularly susceptible to its influence. By blurring the boundaries between advertising and entertainment advertisers may simply overwhelm the defenses children are still in the process of building. (Moore, 2004, p. 165)

In response to the finding that older children are no less susceptible to advertising than younger children, Nairn and Fine (2008) discuss the mechanisms through which marketing influences children. Although much current work focuses on children's cognitive abilities, research in psychology and neuroscience suggests that children's preferences about particular products are shaped by *implicit* attitudes. Such attitudes can be influenced through marketing strategies that are based on "implicit persuasion" and use affective associations to bypass children's explicit understanding of the persuasive intent of advertising. Importantly, changes in implicit attitudes can occur while *explicit* attitudes remain unchanged: "contemporary marketing techniques that link products with positive stimuli can elicit a preference for or choice of that product by non-conscious, non-rational means, and may even undermine consciously held attitudes" (p. 458). This, Nairn and Fine argue, could also explain why *cognitive* defenses—such as the ability to recognize selling or persuasive intent—do not protect older children from the influence of marketing: when marketing strategies bypass cognitive processes, cognitive defenses are not going to be helpful.

This leaves us with a complex picture of the effects of marketing on children, the precise mechanisms through which such marketing operates, and the possible "defenses" children may be building at various stages of their development. Overall, however, there is little disagreement about the fact that children are vulnerable to and affected by the marketing directed toward them. The evidence suggests that children and perhaps even adolescents do not have the same ability to withstand the influence of advertising as adults. How then should policy makers respond to marketing that targets children? The following sections of this chapter consider three possibilities: restricting the extent to which marketing and advertising can reach or attract children; counteradvertising, particularly through social marketing to encourage healthier diets and physical activity; and media literacy education, which aims to help children recognize, critically assess, and resist the content of advertising messages.

Bans on Advertising to Children

The high volume of food advertising targeted at children and its effects on them have led to many calls for restrictions and regulation (e.g., Kelly et al., 2010). Some countries and regions have already adopted restrictions that protect children from advertising to some extent. The most prominent examples of such restrictions occur in Sweden, Ireland, the United Kingdom, and the Canadian province of Québec. Advertising restrictions, of course, tend to meet with strong opposition from the food industry (e.g., Food and Drink Federation, n.d.). As a result, efforts in some areas—for example at the level of the European Union—have focused on appeals to industry self-regulation rather than attempts to directly legislate on the use of marketing techniques targeting children.

However, while self-regulation may be effective in preventing advertisements that are deceptive or misleading, it is not clear how far it can be harnessed for public health purposes. Companies have a collective interest in adverts being seen as nondeceptive, and each individual company has an interest in not being undercut by competitors making extravagant or untruthful claims. By contrast, there are basic discrepancies between the goals of public health and those of private companies, making self-regulation an unlikely tool in the reduction of marketing toward children. Hawkes (2005) emphasizes this point when she explains that

> self-regulation is not designed to ask consumers to *eat less* of their product, use techniques that *less effectively* communicate brand identity, or broadcast *fewer advertisements*. It is usually the contrary. Restricting food advertisements would contravene the manufacturer's goal of promoting greater consumption of what is a perfectly legal, "age-appropriate" product. (p. 381, emphases in original)

As such, self-regulatory organizations are unlikely to commit themselves to creating the kind of media environment that is conducive to healthier choices, so that regulation of food marketing to children becomes necessary (Hawkes, 2005; Moodie et al., 2013; see also Hebden et al., 2011, on the experience with self-regulation in Australia). Indeed, there have been calls for such regulation at the European Union level (Deutsche Welle, 2005).

From a policy perspective, restrictions on advertising may be attractive because studies suggest that they are very cost-effective, relative to other kinds of interventions. Magnus et al. assess the cost-effectiveness of advertising bans with reference to the Australian context. They suggest that, at least in Australia, the cost of enforcing regulation on advertising would be quite low. Indeed, to the extent that improved health outcomes result in lower health care costs, the costs associated with regulation could be fully offset (Magnus et al., 2009). However, the effectiveness of advertising bans remains controversial, especially with companies' ability to move into other channels, such as the Internet, that are more difficult to regulate (Krebs & Schmidt, 2009) and print media, which have received less attention than TV (Jones et al., 2006). We now turn to some issues around implementing such bans and their effects.

Restricting Advertising of Unhealthy Goods to Children: Normative Issues

How should we evaluate the possibility of restricting—or possibly even banning—the advertising of unhealthy food and beverages to children? At first sight, the issues may seem fairly straightforward, ethically speaking. As an especially "impressionable" audience for advertising, children surely deserve special protection from the panoply of sophisticated techniques that marketers have developed to encourage desires that reflect the interests of companies and that have no necessary connection to the needs or interests of consumers. Advertising to children is suspect for at least three reasons. First, children typically lack the resources to interpret and resist advertising messages—pointing to a fundamental inequality between advertiser and consumer that belies standard defenses of advertising as openly persuasive or merely informative. Second, a common argument in favor of free markets—that the consumer is in the best position to balance his or her desires, needs, and interests—does not apply to children, who are not yet in a position to weigh short-term satisfactions against long-term interests. Third, in this domain we have special reasons to think that desires and interests point in opposing directions. As we have noted, sweetened drinks, salty or sugary processed foods, and artificial flavorings and colors readily appeal to children, just as it is in companies' interests to sell highly processed foods based on cheap ingredients. But it is quite clear that there can be "too much of a bad thing" for children.

Of course, companies may argue that it is ultimately parents who make purchasing decisions on behalf of their children: while they market products to children, it is primarily parents who decide what and when to buy. Apart from the fact that children do and must make some purchasing decisions for themselves, this line of thought shows a regrettable—not to say hypocritical—tendency to attribute responsibilities to parents while undermining their power to fulfill those responsibilities. Among parents' many duties is the complex task of helping children understand and act on their own needs, interests, and desires. This task naturally becomes harder to the extent that powerful forces are encouraging children's desires for products that do not serve their needs or interests.

In this context, much has been written about the idea of "pester power." Some authors see the results as akin to a battle between parents and children. Harassed parents are put in a more and more difficult position as the tentacles of marketing—whether directly or via peer pressure among children—intrude into family relations and place strain upon them: "Food marketing aimed at children makes a parent's job harder and undermines parental authority. It forces parents to choose between being the bad guy who says 'no' in order to protect their children's health or giving in to junk-food demands to keep the peace" (Center for Science in the Public Interest, 2003, p. 2). Other authors play down the conflictual element and present the phenomenon as just the latest chapter in a familiar set of disagreements that must be negotiated as part of family life (e.g., Nash & Basini, 2012).

While the balance of evidence speaks to the first view (McDermott et al., 2006), adjudicating between these interpretations is not straightforward—in differing moods and moments, perhaps many parents will be prepared to endorse both views. However, the underlying realities are not really disputable. Children have little economic power, and most purchases of children's food (or toys) will be through parents. Hence effective advertising must encourage children to make effective requests of parents. As we have indicated, this advertising needs to make contact with children's desires, but it has no necessary connection to their needs or interests. Even on the most benign view of pester power, then, it still remains true that the interests of commercial actors are drawn into family dynamics, against the interests of children and the parents who care about them.[3]

At least in the United States, companies have increasingly articulated a second line of defense, by seeking to frame restrictions on advertising as interference with rights to free speech. But the moral and political case for protecting advertising has little basis. Freedom of expression is important because it upholds and expresses citizens' interests in communication and deliberation (Cohen, 1993). Commercial speech, however, does not really contribute to these interests.[4] To the contrary, companies have a legal obligation to ensure profitability in the interests of their shareholders; they have no legal power to take account of moral or civic values when these conflict with profitability. Companies may reasonably ask for a legal framework that allows them to advertise on an equal footing with their competitors. But the fact remains that their advertising is *not* the speech of citizens who are able to consider the public good even when it conflicts with their private interests, and there is no reason to surround it with the protections accorded to individual expression.

---

3. Compare another aspect of marketing—the layout of supermarkets to encourage purchases of sweets by displaying them prominently at checkouts. In a revealing encounter, interviewer James Naughtie challenged Sian Jarvis, corporate affairs director at Asda (UK), about supermarkets' "great displays of fattening and sugar-loaded confectionery to tempt the mother with two children at the checkout." Jarvis rejoined that "one in three of our check outs are guilt free." Instantly spotting Jarvis's flat-footed use of "backstage" language, Naughtie pointed out the implication that two out of three aisles must be "guilty" (because parents either make purchases they believe they should not, or deny their children's wishes). Jarvis's rather feeble defense was that, "We, as retailers, are not there to prevent people making choices about what it is they want to buy" (Stones, 2012).

4. Indeed, there is good evidence that commercial speech is polluting civic discussion by calculated strategies to evade facts or deny scientific findings. Many corporations have gone beyond familiar modes of market competition and engaged in orchestrated attempts, not only to sponsor research that might be favorable to their interests, but actively to undermine research and information sources that seem to interfere with their interests. Such tactics have been well-documented in the case of tobacco, climate change, and chemicals that harm the environment and human health (Union of Concerned Scientists, 2012). Evidently, these alarming developments lie beyond the realm of advertising, in the distortion of scientific research and the manufacture of doubt that far exceeds the normal uncertainties of science and befogs even the clearest scientific findings. ("Doubt is our product," as it was put in one of the more revealing phrases from the tobacco industry's long campaign to suppress evidence about the deadly effects of smoking—see Michaels, 2008.)

Restricting Marketing of Unhealthy Foods to Children: Implementation

Handsley et al. (2009) provide a detailed discussion of possible ways in which advertising restrictions could be structured as well as strengths and limitations of different approaches. First, regulators can focus on *types of programs*. In particular, advertising may be restricted during dedicated children's programs. This is the approach taken in Sweden, where a ban applies to programs "primarily addressed to children under twelve years of age." In the United Kingdom, regulations apply to programs "specifically made for children" and programs "of particular appeal to children." However, as Handsley et al. point out, children may also be exposed to programs for adults, for example when they watch TV with their parents. Advertisements aired during such programs will also attract children's attention. Thus one analysis of the effects of the UK regulations concluded that

> exposure of children to HFSS [high fat, sugar and salt] food advertising, as a proportion of all advertising seen, did not change despite good adherence to the restrictions. . . . By focusing on only a subset of all advertisements that children are exposed to, the UK scheduling restrictions appear to have been flawed from the outset. (Adams et al., 2012, p. 5)

A second approach is to restrict what types of products may be advertised to children. One Australian lobby group advocates a ban on *all* commercial food advertising whenever a significant number of children are watching a particular program (Handsley et al., 2009). However, this may still fail to capture an important aspect of advertising aimed at children: branding of food companies and fast-food chains. As Handsley et al. note, company advertisements may not mention food at all, but campaigns carrying the company's logo and symbols influence children's awareness of that brand, help establish brand loyalty, and encourage children's preferences for that company's food.

An allied approach would be to prohibit the advertising of *unhealthy* foods. This will require agreed-upon definitions of "unhealthy" or "high fat, salt or sugar" foods (Matthews, 2008), which may not be easy to find. And again, such an approach may not capture branding, as fast-food outlets increasingly sell healthier options. Despite these difficulties, however, restrictions on advertising based on the nutritional profile of products give companies an incentive to produce healthier products that *can* be advertised to children. This is, for example, an important aspect of the UK regulations, which are based on the Nutrient Profiling Scheme developed by the Food Standards Agency (Ofcom, 2010). In response to the Ofcom ban, cereal companies have developed products that meet nutritional requirements (Stodell, 2010).

A third possibility is to frame regulatory efforts in terms of the target audience at which particular advertisements are directed. As mentioned above, companies use particular, age-specific techniques to reach children and teenagers. Some regulators therefore prohibit advertisements that are meant to appeal to children. For example, under the restrictions in Québec, "no person may make use of commercial advertising directed at persons under thirteen years of age." To determine whether or not a particular advertisement falls into this category, the regulations refer to "(a) the nature and intended purpose of the goods advertised; (b) the manner of presenting such advertisement; (c) the time and place it is shown" (Handsley et al., 2009). Similarly, in Sweden, advertisements are assessed with respect to their design, the type of product that is advertised, and the context in which they are shown.

Again, however, some kinds of advertisements that attract children's attention to unhealthy foods are likely to fall through the net. Handsley et al. (2009) discuss an advertisement that depicts a young man having a meal at a fast-food restaurant with his child, while watching attractive women eating the chain's salad lunches. Though targeted at adults, the advert also shows a young child enjoying a fast-food meal. Thus regulations that focus on an advertisement's target audience

> have a superficial appeal but are inherently vague and open to interpretation....A regulation applying only to advertising aimed at children is inherently inappropriate and ill-adapted to addressing the contribution of food advertising to childhood obesity.

A fourth strategy is to restrict advertisements shown during particular times of the day. Handsley et al. outline three possibilities here. First, on an "opportunity to watch" approach, we could focus on the structure of children's day to identify when they are available to watch TV. Alternatively, we can use actual viewing patterns, either by focusing on when children make up a certain percentage of the viewing population, or by considering the proportion of children we expect to be watching at any particular time. Such approaches have the advantage of being clearly defined but at the same time, they do not lend themselves to "fine-tuning" in response to changes in the times that children are available to watch TV (e.g., during school breaks) and many relevant advertisements are likely to fall through the net.

A further strategy would be to take note of distinct venues for advertising, and to prohibit it where it is most problematic. At least in the United States, advertising has even entered schools and classrooms: teaching materials are sponsored; vending machines promote foods and drinks; television adverts reach teenagers via Channel One News.[5] In this case, educational institutions become a forum for commercial messages (Brighouse, 2005), bypassing parents' ability to regulate children's viewing or to comment on adverts as they view them with their children. While such intrusion of commerce into schools would not be thinkable in many countries, where it is underway there is an obvious case for regulation to prohibit it.

Finally, regulators can focus on the content of particular advertisements, such as the use of personalities and celebrities that appeal to children (even if the target audience is adults), the use of premiums or give-aways, or strategies that undermine healthy eating. For example, the UK regulations prohibit the suggestion that "having the advertised product somehow confers superiority, for example making a child more confident, clever, popular, or successful," and stipulate that "advertisements should not seem to contradict or ignore good dietary practice" (Ofcom, 2007, pp. 49, 52). Contrast a particularly egregious US advertisement, as described by Joel Bakan (2004):

> Three boys in a school lunchroom excitedly pull bags of chips [crisps] out of their lunch boxes, while a fourth boy, who must make do with only a banana, is unhappy and shunned by the others—at least until he is given a bag of chips, in exchange for his banana, by a monkey. (p. 123)

Bakan goes on to quote industry representatives' appeals to personal and parental responsibility and observes that to make such appeals while deploying these tactics "has more than a ring of hypocrisy about it" (p. 125). As we noted in chapter 3, when commercial actors find themselves committed to incompatible goals, it is a sure sign that regulatory measures are required—notwithstanding companies' inability to admit their need for regulatory intervention.

---

5. See the website of the Campaign for a Commercial Free Childhood (http://commercial-freechildhood.org), last accessed 18 February 2013.

Social Marketing

Social marketing has emerged as one aspect of broader health promotion strategies. There are different definitions of what social marketing is (see Gordon et al., 2006; Kotler et al., 2008), but two features are central. First, social marketing uses techniques from commercial marketing, such as market research, segmentation, and targeting (Gordon et al., 2006; see also Grier & Bryant, 2005; Wong et al., 2004). Second, its objective is the pursuit of social goals. Social marketing aims at voluntary behavior change, by emphasizing the benefits of particular behaviors (Gordon et al., 2006). This can include environmental goals (e.g., to reduce littering) but also social and health problems (Cismaru & Lavack, 2007). Social marketing is explicitly understood by its proponents as a response to commercial marketing techniques and their generally deleterious effects on health-related behaviors: "For decades the health sector has watched as big companies have used marketing to wreak havoc on public health. Social marketing enables us to fight fire with fire" (Hastings & McDermott, 2006, p. 1212). In terms of childhood obesity, there have been prominent campaigns in several countries—for example, the United Kingdom's Change4Life campaign (Department of Health, 2010) and the United States' VERB initiative. Before considering some possible issues raised by social marketing, we first illustrate the broad approach by giving some more detail about VERB, one of the largest of such campaigns.

The VERB campaign, launched in 2002, targeted children between 9 and 13 years of age (and their parents) with the aim of increasing and maintaining physical activity in this group. The intervention phase was preceded by extensive research on children and parents so as to gain an understanding of their behaviors, beliefs, and attitudes (Wong et al., 2004). It used social marketing principles, focusing on the so-called four Ps. The *product* to be promoted was physical activity, which the campaign sought to associate with fun, playing, gaining recognition from peers, and exploring and discovering the world. The *price* refers to costs associated with physical activity, including financial considerations but also psychological, environmental, and time constraints. The aim was to convince parents and children that these costs are outweighed by the benefits of physical activity. Research with the target audience provided insights into how these benefits were viewed by children and their parents. The *place* component emphasized that opportunities for physical activity were readily available.

Finally, as part of the *promotion* component, the VERB campaign had a number of strategies. First, the campaign showed appealing images of physical activity as something for all children. Ads portrayed children from different ethnic backgrounds and also included children with physical disabilities to convey a sense of "kids like me do this" and "I can do that" (Wong et al., 2004). Informed by theories of planned behavior and social cognitive theory, the campaign emphasized the benefits of physical activity (it's social, fun, and cool), self-efficacy ("you don't have to be a pro to be active"), and social influences (many of your peers are having fun being active) (Huhman et al., 2010): "It's all about being 'cool' to their friends and doing what's popular" (Wong et al., 2004, p. 4).

The campaign successfully achieved "brand awareness" but it seems to have had only modest effects on physical activity, as the researchers behind the campaign acknowledge. However, they emphasize that even small changes can add up to significant health benefits: "VERB's positive effects, although modest, are important when viewed in light of the millions of children whose health may be improved" (Huhman et al., 2010, p. 644).

Having set out this example, we now consider some of the issues raised by social marketing campaigns. In the first place, note that social marketing campaigns are often very expensive, and it is not clear that they lead to beneficial outcomes that would justify the expense. The VERB campaign, for example, involved costs of $339 million (approximately €260 million), mainly due to the purchase of prime advertising spots and the use of commercial marketing companies. As indicated, however, it resulted in only modest increases in physical activity. This mirrors wider findings that social marketing tends to have only quite modest effects (Evans, 2006). Decisions to use social marketing should be based on a comparison of expected outcomes with those that could be achieved by alternative uses of resources.

One part of the difficulty here is that social marketing represents a response to the commercial marketing to which people are exposed. Even if social marketers may enjoy greater credibility than commercial advertisers, competing with the marketing efforts of the food and drink industry is clearly an uphill task. The food industry conducts extensive market research to better understand children's food choices and the influence of different marketing strategies on those choices (Nestle, 2006). Further, food companies have vast budgets to finance marketing campaigns for their products; social marketing campaigns, even relatively well-funded ones such as VERB, operate with significantly smaller budgets (Harris et al., 2009b). For example, Randolph and Viswanath (2004) note that in 2002, the McDonald's Corporation spent around $1.3 billion on advertising whereas most social marketing campaigns have smaller budgets than VERB's. They caution that the competitive media environment in which social marketers promote health messages is likely to affect the success of social marketing campaigns.

Another side of the same problem emerges when we consider that social marketing is "pushing against" structural factors that encourage less healthy behaviors. As such, many of the concerns we raised in chapter 6 about individualist approaches to public health apply to the use of social marketing as well. By focusing on individual behavior change, social marketing leaves environmental factors that shape such behaviors out of the picture, or at best suggests ways for individuals to surmount existing barriers. Thus Randolph and Viswanath (2004) point to the importance of environmental factors that enable individuals to make the behavior changes that a campaign promotes: "the success of a mass media campaign in promoting change in a behavior depends on the nature of the environment that will facilitate the change and the structural changes that accompany or are concomitant with campaigns" (p. 426).

The frequent "mismatch" between environments and social marketing messages also gives rise to the worry that such campaigns may contribute to stigmatization of certain groups—a concern that is recognized even in the literature that is positive about social marketing (e.g., Grier & Bryant, 2005). By focusing on individual behavior, campaigns may contribute to judgments of responsibility about, or feelings of culpability among, those who find it hard to adopt the behaviors promoted by particular campaigns (Herrick, 2007). While, to our knowledge, there are no studies that test the effects of such messages on children, a study by Lewis et al. (2010) suggests that obese adults can feel stigmatized by public health messages.

Of course, most advocates of social marketing are well aware of these difficulties. We raise them here not as decisive objections but only to emphasize that social marketing can do relatively little on its own, and is no panacea for the mass marketing—and many other factors—that promotes less healthy behaviors. Nonetheless, social marketing can usefully complement (or promote) other initiatives to prevent childhood obesity and to make environments less obesogenic.

Media Education and Media Literacy

Even when some forms of advertising are regulated, others, such as Internet adverts, are harder to regulate effectively (Krebs & Schmidt, 2009). Furthermore, even if children could be fully isolated from such marketing, they will be exposed to it once they are older. This suggests that we should also be trying to develop children's ability to choose for themselves, for example, by recognizing the ways in which others try to influence their choices (Wickins-Drazilova & Williams, 2011, p. 9f). Media education, which may include critical views on marketing but also a wide range of other topics and skills, is offered in many European countries (Lemmen, 2005). As a response to marketing, media literacy aims to enhance children's ability to recognize and critically reflect on marketing strategies aimed at them.

As such, media literacy may help mitigate some of the possible negative effects of children's and young adults' exposure to the media and help them become critical media consumers and citizens who can make informed choices (Kaiser Family Foundation, 2003). Media literacy education emphasizes a number of principles: that media messages are constructed; that media messages represent reality from particular points of view and with implicit value assumptions; that different media use different rules to construct messages; that individuals interpret media messages based on their own personal experience; and that media are driven by profit within specific economic and political contexts (Kaiser Family Foundation, 2003).

Media literacy has been used in health promotion contexts. Bergsma and Carney (2008) review a range of media literacy interventions, including those targeting nutrition, body image, and eating disorder prevention. For example, media literacy has been used to enhance girls' resistance to powerful media images and messages about women's body shapes (Piran et al., 2000). In the obesity context, media literacy could help children recognize food adverts and the techniques and methods through which particular foods are made to appeal to them. It might also help children negotiate the wider media landscape, which so often—as we stressed in chapter 6—encourages a selective and idealized view of important realities.

Media literacy education could be targeted directly at children, as is (for example) the United Kingdom's MediaSmart program (itself funded by advertisers), which includes materials designed for use in school teaching. Since advertising strategies may work differently with different age groups, "Media literacy programs should be designed to be age-specific, reflecting the differing persuasive techniques effective on children of different ages and teenagers, and the same age-specific considerations should be employed when formulating potential changes to media regulation" (Jones et al., 2006, p. 2116). Similarly, Brand suggests that media literacy education through schools has modest effects but to achieve a greater impact, it is necessary to involve parents and other community members (Brand, 2007).

As noted earlier in this chapter, marketing strategies often work by bypassing explicit beliefs. So there are also reasons to be cautious about media literacy. Greater understanding of the persuasive intent of advertising will not necessarily protect children from its effects (Harris et al., 2009b; Livingstone & Helsper, 2006). Similarly, Bergsma and Carney (2008) note in their review that there is a lack of evidence about the effectiveness of such interventions and inconsistencies in the outcomes measured. These cautions regarding the importance of an evidence-based approach are well-taken, and we must not overestimate how much could be achieved through media literacy education in the obesity context. Nonetheless, it seems to us that developing children's consumer skills, and hence abilities to navigate an "obesogenic" environment, is too important a strategy to neglect, even if we still lack solid evidence concerning the most effective ways to intervene in this regard.

As a final point, we should not forget that parents themselves frequently "mediate" advertising messages. Sometimes this is by restricting children's access to them, but it may also involve explaining the purpose and nature of advertising during or after viewing. In addition, parents actively interpret consumer culture to children, mediating their relation to material goods and controlling their purchases. Studies of these effects by Moniek Buijzen et al. (Buijzen, 2009; Buijzen et al., 2008; Buijzen & Valkenburg, 2005) show that parents' efforts to explain advertising and limit materialism had an important correlation with children's consumption, purchase requests, and conflicts with parents, and "significantly reduced the impact of advertising on children's food consumption" (Buijzen, 2009, p. 105). Similarly, Yu (2011) found that greater interaction while watching television and parental control of television viewing were important factors in reducing children's positive attitudes toward advertising. While it is hard to compare the effects of such mediation with the relatively few attempts to deliberately instill media literacy, it is clear that parents have this opportunity on a daily basis. The active interpretation of adverts and management of consumer culture is surely an important part of the parental role—albeit one that obviously depends on parents' own confidence and understanding of advertising strategies and the market context. As such, interventions may also aim to develop parents' abilities to effectively mediate advertising (e.g., Hindin et al., 2004, p. 194).

Conclusion

As Lang and Rayner put it (2007), "antisocial marketing" is a fact of contemporary life (p. 178). Empirical studies confirm that children are exposed to considerable amounts of marketing for foods high in salt, sugar, and fat, and that such marketing may have significant effects on their food preferences and choices. All the evidence suggests that this encourages increased consumption of such foods, which in turn suggests a link to increased rates of childhood obesity. This presents a formidable challenge to policy makers. In this chapter, we considered several ways in which they might respond. First, bans on adverts targeting children, such as those implemented in the United Kingdom, Sweden, and Québec, may go some way toward protecting children from advertising. It is unlikely, however, that such bans could ever fully isolate them from marketing techniques, especially given the increasing reliance on digital media, which is much harder to regulate than TV advertising. A second strategy is to adopt social marketing campaigns to counter some of the effects of commercial advertising: such campaigns rely on the (often highly successful) methods and techniques of commercial marketers to promote healthy lifestyles. It is clear, however, that social marketers cannot match the funds that companies have available for this. Third, media literacy education could be a promising tool in enhancing children's ability to recognize the persuasive content of marketing campaigns and help them negotiate an environment in which they are bombarded by clever marketing techniques. On their own, all of these approaches are likely to have only modest or uncertain effects. Nonetheless, we would suggest that they can complement each other and be helpful parts of a broader strategy to tackle childhood obesity.

9 SCHOOLS AND CHILDHOOD OBESITY

Schools have been the focus for many interventions to address or prevent weight gain among children. The vast majority of children go to school and spend a substantial part of their day there, and educational institutions facilitate the implementation of health promotion schemes (Haskins et al., 2006; Peterson & Fox, 2007; Story et al., 2006). While some school-based interventions report reductions in BMI (Flodmark et al., 2006; Sahota et al., 2001; Veugelers & Fitzgerald, 2005), commentators have been somewhat disappointed with the effects of school-based interventions on children's body weight or BMI (Cook-Cottone et al., 2009). However, as we emphasized in chapter 2, there are important concerns about the use of BMI, particularly in children, and there are good reasons not to rely on it when assessing interventions. Even if school-based interventions do not lead to clear benefits in terms of weight-based measures, they may improve important health behaviors, such as physical activity or fruit and vegetable consumption (Müller et al., 2005), thus leading to health benefits even if they do not reduce obesity rates (Cook-Cottone et al., 2009).

While school-based obesity interventions may promote some of the goals we want schools to pursue for children, there is also the possibility of conflict. Putting the point at its strongest, Michael Gard and Carolyn Vander Schee argue that using schools to address wider social problems is tokenistic and interferes with schools' basic responsibilities (Gard, 2011a, ch. 5). In this chapter, we consider areas where such conflicts may arise and the extent to which interventions can be worthwhile and conducive to other educational aims. As with the rest of this book, this chapter does not aim to prescribe particular policies for, or uses of, schools. Instead, it explores the main options for intervention and how these might fit with the other responsibilities that schools have.

The most obvious responsibility that schools bear concerns their pupils' education. The next section builds on this truism by setting out three further goals that are also important to the argument of this chapter: children's flourishing and well-being, the development of their autonomy, and equality. The following sections consider two prominent types of school-based anti-obesity interventions—changes to the food environment at school and health education—and explores how they can promote, or come into conflict with, the aforementioned goals of schooling. We then focus on the particular challenge posed by food marketing aimed at children, to which schools have sought to respond in different ways. In the final part of the chapter, we suggest that schools provide an important, if underexplored, opportunity to help protect children from the negative effects of weight stigma, which is an important concern in connection with childhood obesity.

The Goals of Schooling and School-based Obesity Interventions

Much of the philosophical literature on educational goals focuses on highly controversial issues such as religious or citizenship education, which touch on children's ability to choose between different conceptions of the good or the development of their political agency (e.g., Gutmann, 1980; Hand, 2002). However, even seemingly innocuous interventions such as those proposed to combat childhood obesity may come into conflict with the general objectives we want schools to pursue.

One of the most uncontroversial aims of schools is, of course, to educate children. However, this is not simply an end in itself, and many political discussions situate this goal alongside others, such as the development of a skilled workforce. Furthermore, many philosophers stress that this goal needs to be situated in somewhat broader terms. The most widely endorsed of these broader goals include, first, that schools should play an important role in protecting and promoting children's flourishing and well-being; second, that they should further the development of children's autonomy; and, finally, that schools have an important role to play with respect to equality. In this chapter, then, we will consider obesity interventions not just from the perspective of education narrowly understood, but also with attention to the wider aims of developing informed citizens who stand in relations of equality.

Flourishing and Well-being

The idea that schools should further children's well-being and flourishing is common among philosophers (Brighouse, 2008, 2009; Haji & Cuypers,

2008). It also finds echoes in the legal and everyday idea that schools act *in loco parentis*—"in place of a parent"—during the school day. While some elements of what constitutes well-being or flourishing are controversial (see Marples, 2002), there is little dispute that good health is a central aspect of well-being and also facilitates the pursuit of other life goals. An obligation to facilitate children's flourishing must therefore include a commitment to promote their health and physical well-being. In addition, ensuring that children are in good health facilitates the provision of other educational goals: "Health and education success are intertwined: schools cannot achieve their primary mission of education if students are not healthy and fit" (Story et al., 2009, p. 72). Furthermore, some activities that are not always considered educational—such as play time and physical activity—may have positive effects on concentration and academic performance: too narrow a focus on academic education may therefore be self-defeating.

Some obvious features make schools an attractive setting for anti-obesity interventions. Story et al. (2009) note that "schools have an unparalleled opportunity to promote children's health by creating an environment in which children eat healthy foods, engage in regular physical activity, and learn lifelong skills for healthy eating and active living" (pp. 72–73). However, it is not obvious that all such interventions will be compatible with schools' other aims, and some of them may have unintended negative effects, as we consider below.

Autonomy

A second educational goal—the idea that schools should promote or facilitate the development of children's autonomy—is cited frequently in the philosophical literature.[1] While different conceptions of autonomy may come into play here, it is skills and capacities such as the ability to think critically about different conceptions of the good life that are often emphasized. For example, Brighouse (2009) states that "the autonomous person is reflective, and responds to reasons, whether those reasons concern his own well-being or that of others" (p. 37). In other words, schools should help equip children to make their own choices, which includes understanding the context in which one chooses and the effects of one's choices on others.

---

1. This is not an uncontroversial goal; for example, Hand (2006) argues that autonomy is not an appropriate goal for schooling.

In many cases, the choices we make for ourselves will be ones that support our health, and we might hope that school-based activities that encourage healthier lifestyles will always be conducive to autonomy. However, we should remember that autonomous choices may not always be healthy choices. As we have stressed, people aim to balance many different goals as they pursue their lives. Sometimes we decide—often in ways that we would consider autonomous—that the value of health is outweighed by other competing goals. For example, many women decide that, for them, the value of having biological children is worth the health risks involved in pregnancy. If our interest is in individual autonomy, we will want people to critically reflect on their values and the priority they give to health, and then act in accordance with their considered views. This may lead to autonomous decisions to pursue particular goals even if they are not conducive to a person's health. To combine the values of health and autonomy, it is important—especially as children get older—that pupils have opportunities to appreciate the reasons behind school-based interventions. In some cases, it might well be possible and appropriate for them to contribute to decisions about changes to the school environment.

Another aspect of autonomy is also relevant when we are considering health promotion in schools. Responding to concerns about commercialism and the "consumer society," Schinkel et al. (2010) have recently emphasized that autonomy involves developing stable preferences and an ability to make choices consistent with one's long-term interests:[2]

> An autonomous agent…is (ordinarily) someone with a fairly stable set of fundamental concerns and an equally stable preference structure. She is able to make prudent decisions in view of her long-term interests, and not immediately swayed by any internal impulse or external stimulus. (p. 279)

Children, of course, are not yet autonomous agents in this sense. Schinkel et al. (2010) argue that this aspect of autonomy comes under threat in consumer societies, making it difficult for children to develop stable preferences and concerns. With their focus on consumption and materialism, consumer societies "encourage…short-term gratification over long-term interest, impulse over commitment, and they discourage the exercise of self-control" (p. 279).

Related concerns apply in the context of health and childhood obesity. As we discussed in chapter 6, a number of features of the environments that

---

2. In developing this understanding of autonomy, Schinkel et al. draw on Noggle (2002).

characterize contemporary societies have been implicated in the rise in childhood obesity: children are exposed to marketing for unhealthy, energy-dense foods; playing outside is increasingly difficult in areas without appropriate green spaces and playgrounds and in light of concerns about children's safety; and many sedentary behaviors, such as TV and video games, compete for children's time and attention. In such environments, if children "give in" to the desire for immediate enjoyment, this will often result in an unhealthy behavior. In fact, one of the main challenges that stands in the way of healthy choices— not just with respect to children—is that "the costs of most unhealthy activities impact in the future, whereas the benefits from them occur in the present" (Le Grand & Srivastava, 2009). From the points of view of both health and autonomy, a special concern must be to enable children to make appropriate choices within environments in which unhealthy options are often the easiest. Schools, it seems, could make an important contribution to the development of such capacities in children. However, different anti-obesity strategies may not be equally conducive to this goal, as we discuss below.

Equality

Social inequalities in health outcomes have become a central concern in public health and their reduction is now an explicit goal of many interventions. As we discussed in chapter 4, such inequalities have also been observed in childhood obesity in high-income countries, with obesity rates generally being higher in lower socioeconomic and ethnic minority groups (e.g., Due et al., 2009; Saxena et al., 2004). There have been concerns that anti-obesity interventions may be more effective among more advantaged groups and that they could therefore lead to increases in social inequalities (Müller et al., 2005; Swinburn, 2009). This may also apply to interventions in schools.

In addition, schools play a broader role in mediating the social positions to which children eventually gain access and thus their life chances. Admission to a university or attractive occupations often depends on school grades. In many countries, even primary school grades can be crucial because of their importance in gaining access to academically oriented or prestigious secondary schools. Brighouse and Swift (2008) emphasize this important role of the education system as a "gateway" to social positions:

> Modern industrial societies are structured so that socially produced rewards—income, wealth, status, positions in the occupational structure and the opportunities for self-exploration and fulfillment that

come with them—are distributed unequally. Education is a crucial gateway to these rewards; a person's level and kind of educational achievement typically has a major influence on where she will end up in the distribution of those potentially life-enhancing goods. It is unfair, then, if some get a worse education than others because, through no fault of their own, this puts them at a disadvantage in the competition for these unequally distributed goods. (p. 446)

Although educational equality is a controversial ideal that is open to several different interpretations (Brighouse & Swift, 2008, 2009), there is widely shared concern that parents' socioeconomic status often affects children's educational achievement. If the school system is to promote fairness in the competition for desirable positions—or at least not exacerbate any existing unfairness—it therefore needs to support the performance of children who are not already advantaged by their parents' social position. As we suggest below, anti-obesity interventions can affect these mechanisms, particularly through possible effects on academic performance.

Improving Food Environments in Schools

In this and the following sections of this chapter, we will consider different kinds of school-based policy approaches and how they might be conducive to—or come into conflict with—the goals discussed above: to educate children and to promote their well-being and autonomy, as well as equality. We begin by considering school-based initiatives to improve nutrition.

In most countries, children have meals and snacks in schools, and often some or all of this food is provided by the schools (Dixey et al., 1999). As Fox et al. note, this puts schools in "a unique position to influence children's food choices on a daily basis and potentially contribute to development of healthful dietary habits and preferences—no other institution has as much continuous and intensive contact with children" (Fox et al., 2009, p. S57). Improving such meals is an integral part of many school-based interventions. The provision of healthy food also ensures that what children eat at school is consistent with what they learn about healthy eating in the classroom (Finkelstein et al., 2004). Many interventions thus aim to improve the nutritional value of meals provided in schools; to discourage the sale of foods high in fat, salt, or sugar; and to increase the consumption of healthier options, such as fruits and vegetables. For example, the provision of free fruit has been found to increase—at least in the short term—fruit consumption among children (Te Velde et al., 2008). A German study that provided primary schools with water fountains and integrated lessons on the importance of drinking water into the curriculum led to lower obesity compared to the control schools (Muckelbauer et al., 2009).

While many interventions increase the availability of healthier foods without restricting access to unhealthy options, a different strategy is to limit children's access to unhealthy foods. This includes, first, "competitive foods" (i.e., foods offered outside of schools' meal programs), which have been a target in many school-based interventions. Especially in the United States, vending machines and à la carte menus are a source of unhealthy meals, snacks, and drinks (Veugelers & Fitzgerald, 2005). Interventions may require that vending machines no longer provide sugary drinks, or that à la carte menus meet certain nutritional requirements. Second, some initiatives have focused on the foods children bring into the school, for example by attempting to improve the packed lunches parents provide for their children or by putting restrictions on what foods can be brought to school.

Can such policies contribute to the educational goals we have mentioned? Schools' most obvious goal of educating children could arguably be promoted by these initiatives. As we mentioned above, such policies can help ensure that schools' food environment is consistent with what children learn about healthy nutrition as part of the curriculum. Gross discrepancies between educational messages and school foods undermine messages about healthy nutrition. Healthier food environments, on the other hand, support such messages and ensure that concepts of healthy eating do not remain abstract concepts, but become a matter of experiential learning. Engaging children in the decision-making process in some way could further bring home the importance of healthy nutrition, in line with the information children are receiving in class.

What about the broader goals we discussed in the previous section? Consider first well-being. The main argument presented in favor of policies to improve the food environment in schools is that they could contribute to pupils' health. Some commentators suggest that the evidence on the association between the availability of competitive foods and students' weight is not clear-cut (Minaker et al., 2011). However, if it is true that consumption of healthier options, particularly fruits and vegetables, is beneficial for children's health even in the absence of weight loss, it is not necessary to require that the connection between these policies and the reduction or prevention of overweight and obesity is fully established; it would be sufficient for there be a move toward the consumption of healthier foods. Here, too, however, the evidence is not clear-cut. Although some studies suggest that the availability of unhealthy competitive foods increases children's consumption of such foods and may replace consumption of healthier options, particularly fruits and vegetables (Cullen et al., 2006), it has also been suggested that restrictions on competitive foods do not necessarily reduce their consumption, as children simply rely on sources outside school. For example, one study suggested that students seemed to respond to the reduced availability of sugar-sweetened beverages in the school by bringing such drinks from home or increasing consumption outside of school (Cullen et al., 2006). In other studies, reducing the availability of sugar-sweetened beverages in schools did not lead to lower consumption of such beverages (Taber et al., 2012; Whatley Blum et al., 2008).

There may also be a cost to this kind of restrictive policy in terms of the development of children's and young adults' autonomy. Food environments outside of schools tend to offer a wide array of unhealthy food options. In the absence of radical policy changes to alter these environments, children find themselves surrounded by these options when they leave school, both at the end of the school day and later in life. As we discussed above, an important aspect of autonomy is that children learn how to evaluate the options available to them in terms of their preferences, values, and long-term interests; that they can understand how it is that they come to be presented with a given range of options; and that they can follow through on the decisions they eventually make.

Is a restrictive approach to the kinds of food available in schools conducive to this objective? This is, at least to some extent, an empirical question. Schinkel et al. (2010) suggest that, with respect to the influence of commercialism, schools can help develop children's autonomy by providing an environment in which they are protected from the most problematic aspects of consumer societies: "pupils need at least a space in which they are free from those influences and preferably one in which they are offered the opportunity to develop temporally extended agency" (p. 282). There is, however, a possible tension here. On the one hand, protecting children from the influence of consumer societies means that they may miss out on opportunities to "practice" relevant skills, such as turning down unhealthy options when such options are available.[3] On the other hand, ensuring a healthy diet in school

---

3. Note that this point is different from the objection that restricting children's choices for their own good is problematic. Children, especially those at young ages, are not yet in a position to make fully autonomous choices. Interfering with such choices for the children's benefit clearly may be considered paternalist; but given children's limited capacity for choice,

may allow children to become accustomed to, and develop preferences for, certain kinds of food and pave the way for healthy food patterns in other, less restrictive, environments. The strength of these competing considerations may vary for children at different ages. At younger ages, when children's food preferences are being shaped and they cannot distinguish between healthy and unhealthy foods, it may be beneficial to remove unhealthy options. Once children become older, however, removing unhealthy foods may be counter-productive, as they will have access to such foods outside school and must develop the skills necessary to make sensible choices as consumers. There may also be important benefits to be gained from involving children—especially older ones—in the decision about what kinds of food and drink are available in schools. This would address children as future citizens participating in col-lective decisions that strike a balance between competing considerations and opinions. Empirical research could help us assess the extent to which these different mechanisms come into play.

Tensions can also emerge when we consider anti-obesity interventions from the perspective of equality. First, interventions may turn out to be more beneficial for children from better-off backgrounds than they are for those from poorer families; such effects could heighten social inequalities in health. For example, some interventions that aim to improve the food children con-sume in school focus not on what institutions provide but on items children bring from home, as packed lunches and snacks have been found to be a source of unhealthy food. In a study from the United Kingdom, researchers found that only 1.1 percent of the packed lunches they examined met all nutritional requirements that apply to English school meals (Evans et al., 2010). They designed an intervention that provided parents with lunch boxes and refill-able water bottles and gave them information about what foods to include in their children's lunches. Their low cost may make such interventions worth-while, even though the authors of the study find only modest improvements in the quality of packed lunches. Further, since the policy was rolled out universally, it did not appear to stigmatize overweight children (Cuttini & Barreto, 2010), making it compatible with schools' commitment to protect children's emotional well-being. However, the study did not assess whether it was effective with parents from disadvantaged backgrounds, whose ability to

---

paternalist intervention is what is required in many contexts; see our discussion in chapter 6, section "Paternalism and the Interests of Parents and Children." The point is only that we need to think carefully about which strategy will best enable children to choose healthy foods as they grow up to become choosers and consumers in their own right.

provide nutritious food for their children may be restricted by financial and time constraints. This question is, however, crucial in assessing whether or not this intervention may come into conflict with concerns about equality.

School-based obesity interventions may also affect broader concerns about equality of opportunity, in particular because of possible effects of such interventions on academic performance. On the one hand, school-based interventions could make an important contribution to social equality by addressing some of the factors that disadvantage children from poorer backgrounds. In particular, school-based interventions may help address social inequalities in children's access to healthy foods. Similarly, students from lower income backgrounds are less likely to have nutritious breakfasts than children from more affluent families (O'Dea & Wilson, 2006). Since regular breakfast appears to improve concentration and academic performance (Rampersaud et al., 2005), ensuring provision of a healthy breakfast in schools could help level the playing field.[4]

However, it is not clear that such interventions lead to equal benefits for students from different backgrounds. A study of UK chef Jamie Oliver's initiatives that aimed to improve food provided in several London schools suggests that affluent children's educational outcomes improved as a result of healthier school meals but less so, or not at all, for children from poorer backgrounds (Belot & James, 2011). This is particularly problematic once we consider that, with school performance, what matters is often not just how well children are doing in absolute terms, but also how their performance compares to that of other children. If changes in school meals increase the performance gap, this will make it even harder for children from disadvantaged backgrounds to compete for the kinds of goods and opportunities that schools provide access to, even if their grades do not become worse in absolute terms. The finding from London is, of course, only preliminary and may not hold for other interventions. However, these effects are generally not measured in school-based interventions. Making such considerations part of the assessment and evaluation of school-based interventions could assist the design of policies that are conducive to, rather than problematic for, the pursuit of equality.

Finally, we should also take account of interventions' possible effects on social equality more broadly. For example, after the introduction of the

---

4. Eating breakfast regularly also appears to help prevent obesity (Davis et al., 2007, p. S232; Quick et al., 2013), although some authors argue that a definite case has not yet been made (Casazza et al., 2013, p. 450).

Schools Health Promotion and Nutrition Scotland Act, some Scottish schools banned birthday cakes and bake sales (Horne, 2010). Such bans are, of course, controversial, and may even be counterproductive insofar as they place home-cooked products in the same category as processed foods. In addition, regulating what parents can give their children to consume raises difficult questions about the appropriate scope of parental authority. Parents may well regard the provision of food as central to parenting and as a way of expressing care and affection toward their children. For example, one study found that mothers regarded feeding their children as "an important and emotionally rewarding part of parenting that [they] seemed unwilling to relinquish" (Jain et al., 2001, p. 1140). Furthermore, interference with parental choices in this context may also be taken to express an implicit understanding that parents cannot be trusted to feed their children an appropriate diet, thus contributing to the stigmatization of the (often already disadvantaged) parents of over-weight children.

These concerns suggest that we must consider the broader effects of obesity interventions on different aspects of equality. Interventions that aim to improve food provided by or consumed in schools may improve children's well-being but may not mesh smoothly with the development of children's autonomy and considerations of equality.

Health Education: Knowledge and Practical Skills

The second type of anti-obesity intervention we consider concerns health education, broadly conceived. The provision of knowledge that will promote children's health is often regarded as an integral component of teaching children how to look after themselves and of preparing them for adulthood (Brooks & Magnusson, 2010). Providing children at different ages with information about what constitutes healthy nutrition is an important aspect of school-based interventions and indeed can be argued to represent a basic aspect of education.

The provision of such information can help children make informed choices about food and nutrition, thus making a contribution to the kind of autonomy discussed above. Furthermore, this kind of intervention could also be important from the perspective of equality: it has been suggested that food knowledge is better among children from advantaged backgrounds (in terms of income or education) relative to those from disadvantaged backgrounds (Gwozdz & Reisch, 2011; Sichert-Hellert et al., 2011). Ensuring that children gain an understanding of what healthy nutrition involves could help even out some of these differences between children from different socioeconomic groups. The empirical evidence, however, suggests that such interventions may sometimes be detrimental to equality. An Irish study found that the introduction of nutrition education in primary schools appeared to have a smaller impact on schools in deprived areas compared to those in more affluent neighborhoods (Friel et al., 1999).

Furthermore, there are concerns about possible negative effects that nutrition education could have on children's well-being. First, critics argue that the information conveyed through nutrition lessons may have negative effects on students. It may inadvertently encourage unsupervised weight-loss attempts, which can lead to growth failure, height stunting, or reduced bone density (O'Dea, 2010), and contribute to the use of unhealthy weight-loss techniques such as starvation, vomiting, laxative abuse, diuretic and diet pill usage, and cigarette smoking to suppress appetite (Strauss & Mir, 2001). Nutrition education that focuses on weight and weight control may also contribute to body image concerns among young people (O'Dea, 2010). Many studies do not explicitly evaluate to what extent such problems arise, so it is difficult to gauge how common or significant such effects are. However, since we know that these are already significant and widespread problems, at least in older children (Larson et al., 2009; Neumark-Sztainer et al., 2011; Neumark-Sztainer et al., 2012), it makes good sense for interventions and educational measures to address these issues and to counter the misconception that weight loss is necessarily beneficial to health.

Nutrition education need not be restricted to the provision of information about healthy food and promoting children's understanding of healthy nutrition. Commentators have suggested that health education should involve the acquisition of more practical skills. For example, Lichtenstein and Ludwig suggest that the reintroduction of home economics into the school curriculum could help address obesity (Lichtenstein & Ludwig, 2010). They describe this as a practical, skills-oriented subject that could teach children basic cooking techniques, budget principles, food safety, and how to find and use nutrition information. Such an approach would seem to make an important contribution to developing children's autonomy, by strengthening their ability to make better-informed food purchase decisions and making them less dependent on food prepared by others. Furthermore, with respect to equality, this kind of approach could be particularly helpful in reaching children from disadvantaged backgrounds, who often face multiple barriers in adopting healthier behaviors.

However, it is crucial that we select appropriate skills to be taught to children in this context; not all skills will be conducive to children's emotional and physical well-being. One obesity prevention program implemented in a primary school provided children with advice on how to reduce feelings of hunger, for example by brushing teeth right after eating, having soup before their meal, or eating low-calorie foods first (Jiang et al., 2007). While such practical advice may benefit obese children and adolescents who are having difficulty controlling their eating, advising children how to "trick" hunger cues and emphasizing weight loss is, of course, hugely problematic and may run counter to the pursuit of children's well-being. The narrow focus on weight outcomes that is common to many studies can obscure the broader effects of such interventions.

Finally, education about nutrition can be looked at in broader terms, regarding food culture, availability, and systems. In general, a crucial task of education is to enable children to begin to explore and appreciate the complex systems on which modern societies depend. As we discussed in chapter 6, modern systems of food production have created an almost total divorce between farm, factory, and consumer. Many programs have been introduced so that children can learn more about where their food comes from, such as practical initiatives to grow food on school grounds, or to develop relations with local farms and build educational and food supply links with them. These are relevant to children even in the first years of school.[5] For older children, such initiatives can be supplemented and developed by more academic treatment of the many dimensions of modern agriculture and food supply systems, in subjects such as biology, chemistry, economics, geography, and history. Of course, such measures are unlikely, by themselves, to generate clear reductions in childhood obesity or improvements in health. But they promise other significant benefits—above all, citizens who better understand the real cost and value of food and can appreciate the important societal issues bound up with nutrition and health.

Responding to Food Marketing Aimed at Children

The marketing of unhealthy foods to children has been identified as an important problem in the context of childhood obesity. We discussed this issue— and possible responses to it—in chapter 8; here we briefly comment on its

---

5. For example, see the Food for Life Partnership—online at http://www.foodforlife.org.uk.

relevance in schools and the goals of schooling that we focused on in this chapter. Given schools' investment in children's well-being, responding to the increasing presence of adverts for food (and other products) in children's lives seems warranted. Exposure to food advertising seems to result in greater consumption of unhealthy food and has been linked to worse health in children (Cairns et al., 2009). There are also broader concerns that children's exposure to advertising could lower their well-being and self-esteem (Buijzen, 2003; Nairn et al., 2007). Studies also suggest that children and adolescents are concerned about the symbolic aspects of particular brands and what they want to be *seen* to eat in settings—such as school—where they interact with peers (Stead et al., 2011). Furthermore, interventions that succeed in protecting children from the effects of advertising can provide benefits from the perspective of equality: studies suggest that children from low-income backgrounds are more exposed to marketing than are children in higher income families (Kumanyika & Grier, 2006).

Unfortunately, it is far from clear which approaches best protect children from marketing. As in the case of interventions targeting the food environment, the tensions inherent in identifying an effective response to advertising become particularly apparent in relation to the goal of autonomy. Schools may seek to ban marketing practices from the school environment. The presence of marketing in schools can be particularly problematic as it may be taken to legitimate the practice of targeted advertising and imply that the products advertised are condoned or supported by the schools. Limiting the degree to which companies can use the school environment to advertise their products may shield children from these effects to some extent.

Nonetheless, even if schools are fully isolated from advertising practices, children will be exposed to food marketing outside the school environment. As we discussed in chapter 8, only a small number of regions and countries have put in place legislation to protect children from the effects of marketing. Even then, limitations of regulation and the intractability of channels such as the Internet mean that children are exposed to advertising (Kent et al., 2011; Krebs & Schmidt, 2009). As we considered in chapter 8, companies have developed a multitude of effective ways of reaching their target audiences. Therefore attempts to increase children's resilience to such marketing may also be beneficial. Some commentators have expressed doubt about the potential of media literacy interventions in protecting children from marketing techniques, pointing to the powerful impact that marketing has on children and the vast amounts of emotional and often very subtle advertising to which they are exposed (Harris et al., 2009b). At the same time, these are exactly the kind of mechanisms we normally think of as undermining individual autonomy. Developing abilities to recognize such attempts and the various ways in which corporations attempt to influence their choices would be valuable to children's autonomy and their future health and well-being. While it remains unclear how far it is possible to do this, we would suggest that the strategy of developing children's ability to navigate this particular aspect of the obesogenic environment is too important to neglect.

Protecting Children from the Effects of Weight Stigma and Weight-based Teasing

The previous sections considered some of the most prominent school-based anti-obesity interventions: changes to the food environment, health and nutrition education, and responses to food marketing targeting children. This section considers efforts that have received much less attention in the obesity context: interventions that aim to challenge weight-based stigma. Clearly, there are many reasons why schools should attempt to combat all forms of discrimination and bullying, not least in terms of their responsibilities regarding children's well-being. If we are concerned about the effects of childhood obesity, it is crucial to include weight-based teasing and stigma among the list of "targets." Interventions that can tackle weight-based stigma could help protect not only overweight and obese children but also children of "normal" or low weight from psychological harm. Interventions that strengthen children's resilience to weight-based teasing or other forms of stigma may also be beneficial from the perspective of autonomy. Finally, given possible connections between weight stigma and academic performance, such efforts could also be relevant from the perspective of equality.

The psychological harms experienced by overweight or obese children are sometimes presented as if they were a direct or natural consequence of higher body weight. Nonetheless, such harms are clearly mediated by children's and adults' attitudes toward fatter persons, and obese children's experience of stigma is an important factor in the connections between obesity and psychological outcomes (Latner & Schwartz, 2005). The experience of weight-based teasing may lead to anxiety, low self-esteem, and depression (Libbey et al., 2008) and may also have long-term consequences for children's well-being (Eisenberg et al., 2006). Weight-based teasing has been associated with disordered eating behaviors (Libbey et al., 2008; Neumark-Sztainer et al., 2002), and concerns about weight-based stigma and body image may also interfere with the adoption of health behaviors, most notably physical activity (Faith et al., 2002). Studies with adults even suggest that it is the experience of stigma that leads to some of the poorer *physical* health among obese individuals (Muennig et al., 2008; Muennig, 2008). Challenging weight bias and stigmatization may lead to significant benefits for children subject to such stigmatization or weight-based teasing (Puhl & Latner, 2007). Importantly, it is not only obese children who may be subject to weight-based teasing; in one study, underweight children and those of average weight also reported being teased about their weight (Neumark-Sztainer et al., 2002). Interventions that reduce children's exposure to weight-based stigma, or strengthen their ability to cope with or effectively challenge this experience, could make an important contribution to their well-being.

From the perspective of autonomy, too, interventions that strengthen children's ability to maintain self-esteem in the face of weight stigma could be important. For example, one intervention for primary school children used a puppet play to increase children's healthy self-concept and healthy attitudes toward food and eating (Irving, 2000). In a different study, children produced a play in which they reflected on their own experiences of teasing, and also worked with school staff to help them identify their own attitudes toward weight and to learn about how to maintain a healthy body image (Haines et al., 2006). One problem we noted in chapter 5 is that teachers may share antifat attitudes and display negative attitudes toward obese or overweight children. These attitudes must be addressed so that schools can provide a setting in which all children are respected and such initiatives can be implemented.

Finally, weight stigma may also interfere with schools' goals with respect to equality. Negative stereotypes about obese children seem to have negative effects on their academic performance. Some studies suggest that obese children are more likely to be regarded as "stupid" than thin children (Puhl & Latner, 2007), and that such stereotypes have an impact on how children perform in school. Social psychologists have found evidence of the so-called stereotype threat: when individuals who are the target of a negative group stereotype are in a situation where their actions might confirm this stereotype, their performance is likely to be poorer than it would be in the absence of the stereotype threat. In experiments involving standardized tests, for example, participants from lower class backgrounds performed worse than participants from higher class backgrounds when the test was presented as a measure of verbal ability; when the test was not presented as a measure of ability, performance of lower class participants matched that of the higher-class participants (Croizet & Claire, 1998). Similar findings were made with respect to the performance of African Americans (Steele & Aronson, 1995) and women (Spencer et al., 1999). Although it has been suggested that stereotype threat could also be salient for overweight and obese children with respect to general academic performance (Gable et al., 2008), we were unable to find any studies testing these effects in relation to overweight children or adults. One study also suggests that weight-based teasing may play a role in explaining the lower academic performance of overweight children (Krukowski et al., 2009). Whatever the explanation for lower educational outcomes among overweight and obese children, they leave them at a severe disadvantage relative to their thinner peers—and weight stigma may well play an important mediating role.

Conclusion

Growing concerns about the prevalence of childhood obesity have led to increased calls for school-based interventions to tackle obesity among children. Schools, it has been suggested, "may be one of the most important settings in which to promote and sustain healthful nutrition and physical activity" among young people (Bauer et al., 2004, p. 43). This hope may be overstated, since most school-based interventions promise only modest or indirect effects, and obesity prevention is clearly not the principal responsibility that schools should undertake. However, we have argued in this chapter that limited measures to tackle childhood obesity can be compatible both with schools' responsibility to educate and their more diffuse responsibilities to promote children's well-being, autonomy, and equality. As with many other measures proposed to tackle childhood obesity, we should not expect school-based interventions to have immediate or even direct effects on rates of overweight or obesity. At the same time, where interventions promise benefits in other dimensions—such as the broader goals of schooling that we have stressed in this chapter—and prove compatible with existing responsibilities, there may be good reasons to pursue them, especially where their costs and opportunity costs are modest. Of course, not all interventions will pass these tests: caution is needed to avoid tokenistic or otherwise unhelpful measures; and empirical studies and careful evaluation—taking account of effects on many different dimensions—will remain necessary to judge which interventions are really worthwhile.

CONCLUSION

CHILDHOOD OBESITY: SOME PRACTICAL IMPLICATIONS

This book has emphasized complexity rather than simplicity. This is because obesity only *seems* simple. It is also because many different social concerns cluster around childhood and health. Above all, it is because complex problems lack simple solutions.

As we stressed in the book's introduction, we have not asked directly who should do what in order to address childhood obesity. In fact, our simplest prescription has just been the need to appreciate the complexity of the problems, in both ethical and policy terms. Childhood obesity attracts justifiable concern because it is causally related to many serious and chronic health problems. But the causal connections are not simple or fully understood. More than this, we must appreciate that many of the factors that cause obesity also pose dangers to health in those who do not become overweight or obese. Those who are not overweight or obese may be unfit, have poor diets, and suffer from metabolic syndrome. Perhaps oddly in a book about childhood obesity, we have cautioned against making obesity the center of moral concern and social policy. We should be worrying about patterns of behavior—such as low levels of physical activity—and much larger structural issues—such as our systems of food production and processing—that pose risks of ill-health in children and adults, regardless of their weight status. We should also be worried by the fact that stigma, social isolation, and low self-esteem cause misery and even ill-health in many fatter children and adults—and even in some of "normal" weight—regardless of whether their body fat or lifestyles pose particular health risks.

Partly for these reasons, we must resist the promise of simple solutions. In children as in adults, obesity is closely connected to many complex changes in our environments that cannot be simply reversed. Many of those changes—for instance, a situation of food plenty rather than food scarcity—have also led to widespread improvements in health and life expectancy. This fact relates to one structural reason why it is hard to decide what to do about childhood obesity. Not only do we need to address obesity, related health issues, and stigma and discrimination. There are also many other tasks and issues that we need to address. As individuals deciding how to lead our lives, we need to take account of many factors other than health. As societies, we need to engage in wider political debate, so that we can reach decisions that balance our many priorities and make acceptable trade-offs between various costs and benefits. We have also emphasized a second structural reason why it is so hard to give concrete prescriptions. How are we to divide responsibility for action among many different actors who each have other, pre-existing rights and responsibilities? Parents already have many different tasks on their plates; companies already have a legal responsibility to ensure profitability that trumps any other goal; local, national, and federal governments already have many challenging responsibilities. Even if we could agree on the relative priority of obesity interventions, this would not give a simple answer to the question as to who should "step up" and how they should act.

In other words, deciding who should do what raises questions that reach far beyond the scope of a book on childhood obesity. Yet discussions of ethics and policy are ultimately practical in nature: they concern what ought to be done. In this conclusion, then, we would like to summarize some of the positions we have taken in this book and draw out some implications for action that we believe follow from our discussions.

In the first place, because childhood (and adult) obesity is caught up with such complex systems, we have made a negative argument. Measures that promise to address childhood obesity directly may well seem attractive but prove less satisfactory on closer examination. As examples, we mentioned child-measuring programs and social marketing campaigns.

Both the United Kingdom and United States have seen programs to measure all children and send home reports of their weight status. We argued in chapter 2 that this is a simple-minded response. The likely benefits of such policies evaporate on closer examination, while other dangers become apparent—for example, encouraging unhealthy weight loss, focusing attention on children whose weight is already painfully visible, and ignoring much wider patterns of physical unfitness and poor diet. There are much better uses of schools' time and resources than this—not least, as we suggested above, to counter weight-based stigma and bullying.

Child measuring programs also tend to overemphasize parental responsibilities—obviously there is no point in informing parents about their child's BMI status unless parents are meant to act on that information. As we argued in chapter 3, any measure that focuses mainly on parental responsibilities is problematic. A small minority of parents may be failing to do their best by their children, but that minority is largely beyond the reach of anything but highly targeted and resource-intensive interventions. While those may be worthwhile, childhood obesity is just one of the issues that such interventions should take account of. In any event, most parents are already doing the best that they can to negotiate many competing priorities. Encouraging them— let alone hectoring them—to try harder in various ways is both unfair and unlikely to have significant effects. All sorts of complex social and economic shifts have undermined a division of responsibilities that adequately supports parents. There may not be simple ways to address this, but placing greater pressure on parents will do little to help.

Social marketing measures that promote key health messages and encourage healthier behaviors may seem less problematic. We agree that there is a clear role for such measures. This is especially true where a health message is not widely known—as appears to be the case in some countries with regard to adequate sleep time for children, for example. However, we have also pointed out that campaigns marketing health messages are not entirely innocent. One problem is that, in prioritizing health, they tend to instrumentalize food and exercise. As a result, they can detract from the sociability and cultural value that lies in enjoying food together (Fischler, 2011; Food Ethics Council, 2005) or the unadorned pleasures of outdoor play and exploration for children. Again, the wider problem is that, almost unavoidably, they emphasize individual responsibilities and so raise the problem of fairness we have just mentioned. It is much easier to aim messages at individuals and parents than it is to deal with institutional factors such as the quality of school meals, the marketing of foods and drinks in schools, or wider commercial forces and built environments. But it can be very hard for individuals and parents to change their behavior in the face of structural forces that make healthy choices costly or difficult. Hence social marketing for health faces the same dual problem of unfairness and relative ineffectiveness as measures that focus on parental responsibilities.

Turning now to some positive cases for action, we first want to emphasize one goal that we believe is unambiguously worthwhile—the elimination of fat stigma. Although it is difficult to translate into concrete responsibilities, this goal is almost unique in that it does not involve making trade-offs with other important values or goods. As we stressed in chapter 5, our societies are not simply benevolent associations concerned about health and welfare: they also make fat people—including fat children—into objects of shame and ridicule. There is, we believe, every reason to try and reduce our cultural preoccupation with the slim or muscular body and to challenge our cultural distaste for the fat body. These obsessions hurt adults and children alike, in the form of stigma, discrimination, bullying, self-hatred, restricted nutrition, and disordered eating. We believe that there is no goal of social policy, nor anything valuable in our individual lives, that would be damaged were we to abandon the prejudices that cause these tragic consequences. The more we can find ways to stop passing such attitudes onto our children, the better.[1] This might be through antibullying policies that tackle the exclusion and denigration of fatter children or by encouraging children's confidence in their bodies, for example through the enjoyment of physical activity; it might require us to discipline our own urges to diet, to pathologize "fat" or "carbs," and to obsess about our figures. While governments can do relatively little to this end, there is much that parents, schools, and companies can do. Partly for this reason, we have argued that it is important to keep health, not weight, at the center of our concerns.

By contrast, few of the other issues involved with childhood obesity can be addressed without costs or at least challenges to other things that we value. This means that difficult questions of priorities and trade-offs constantly arise. Food production represents a key example. Western governments have promoted and funded industrial agriculture in the name of cheap, secure, and plentiful food supplies. In doing so, they have created a powerful social expectation: most of us do not need to think about where our food comes from, and we do not need to sacrifice other goods in order to afford it. Any change to this system is likely to detract from the cheapness, choice, convenience, plenty, and (dare we say it) thoughtlessness that consumers currently enjoy. It is also likely to damage the interests of powerful economic actors—very large commodity farming concerns; transnational manufacturers of processed foods who depend on cheap commodity agriculture; and supermarkets, whose astonishingly variegated (and tempting!) product ranges depend on the resulting network. Although the results are less than optimal in terms of nutrition and obesity, perhaps some would choose to keep our current systems in place if these were the only issues at stake. Taking questions of sustainability into account too, however, we believe there is an urgent case for action.[2] Nonetheless, this does not alter the fact that any changes will involve losses as well as gains.

---

1. Hence we strongly endorse Berg's emphasis on "the six major weight and eating problems: overweight, eating disorders, dysfunctional eating, undernutrition, hazardous weight loss, and size prejudice" in her book, *Underage and Overweight* (2005, p. 321).

2. For further discussion, see Lang et al. (2009); Lawrence (2008); and Roberts (2008).

As we stressed in chapter 6, it is hard to face these trade-offs head on. One reason is the problem we already mentioned—there are no simple answers as to who should do what. While there is, we believe, a clear political responsibility to regulate this system to promote healthier produce and healthier products—and to reduce its environmental damage and wastefulness—even that responsibility is awkwardly divided between citizens and commerce and politicians, such that changes are hard to initiate and each set of actors can always blame another. Another reason it is hard to face these trade-offs lies in the fact that consumers rarely glimpse the systems that determine the choices open to them. Costs and risks become visible only in occasional moments of crisis, while companies work continuously to promote the benefits that are available to us. Their idealizations and our aspirations work together to obscure the problems in our present systems. These factors make trade-offs look more painful, and changes harder to conceive, than need be.

Similar points apply with regard to physical activity and transport systems. As we know, there are many ways in which contemporary arrangements encourage sedentary behavior and discourage active transport such as cycling and walking. There are many complex institutional responsibilities involved here—in architecture and urban and road planning, for example—to alter built environments so that physical activity plays a larger role in our everyday lives. Those issues have been largely beyond our scope. However, we have stressed that children's needs are often different from adults', so that measures that make neighborhoods friendlier to adults' physical activity may not help children. In addition, increasing perceptions of danger to children too often limit their freedom. Those perceptions are not always realistic, and the urge to protect can itself be dangerous, since children need to develop capacities to navigate risk and take responsibility for themselves. Against this background, we should be cautious of widespread expectations that parents supervise their children at all times. Rather, we believe that legitimate concern with children's safety should be channeled into collective arrangements that promote this. This is no easy task in societies of strangers and busy roads. But there are many strategies for better urban planning that can promote safety through mutual visibility, increased foot and cycle traffic, and reduced vehicle flows. Above all, there are very strong reasons to make the attempt, so that our children can—as our parents mostly did when they were growing up—make their own way to school and spend time being active together without specific adult supervision. Again, it should be noted that such attempts are supported by other considerations, such as the dangers of relying on oil-based energy, including the climate destabilization that anyhow threatens our children's future well-being.

In chapters 7 and 8, we discussed some of the issues around proposals to tax or subsidize certain foods and to deal with marketing by food companies. In terms of tax and subsidy, our main claim was that—before advocating yet another layer of intervention—it is vital to understand the ways in which public policies and public expenditures are already bound up with food production systems. Proposals to tax some foods in certain ways may have merits, but they lack coherence if governments are also subsidizing those same foods, or if their regulatory systems are inept. Hidden from public scrutiny, agricultural subsidies and poor regulation persist partly by inertia and partly because they support powerful constituencies. While tax proposals inevitably raise wider political questions about the role of the state, we have suggested they are especially valuable as provocations. Although there are many arguments to consider against such measures, proposals such as a "soda tax" nonetheless raise questions: How are we going to reduce children's exposure to high-calorie, nonsatiating, nutrient-poor foods and drinks? How *can* governments reform their budgetary and regulatory food policies, which presently favor larger companies and food processors? How can we address the relatively high cost of fresh fruit, vegetables, and unprocessed foods—something that clearly poses special problems for poorer parents?

With regard to food marketing, we believe there is a clear case for protecting children from the most blatant commercial pressures—be they advertisements or product placement in children's television, marketing deals in schools, or the many innovative ways in which the food industry has exploited new communication technologies. But these measures also have something of the character of a rear-guard action. Food companies have shown no will to responsibility and have evaded the spirit if not letter of every regulation, be it "voluntary" or statutory. In addition, children need to learn how to deal with commercial pressures as they grow up. Just as important, then, are the different ways in which we can help children to become savvy consumers, able to decode adverts and branding, with their aspirational messages about identity, status, and lifestyle and their idealized pictures of mundane and often frankly unsatisfying products. Here it is much more difficult to create large-scale policies. Moreover, most adults are in some degree susceptible to the sophisticated and well-funded efforts of marketing professionals, and this naturally limits their ability to mediate the effects of advertising to children. We believe this represents a vital area for social experimentation, especially in the educational system.

Underlying the structural challenges of food and transport systems, taxation and subsidy regimes, and the regulation of marketing are broader questions of state power and its proper scope. We have not taken a strong position on these questions, but we have sought to resist some simpler arguments that dispute the state's role in these spheres. Above all, it is important to appreciate how far-reaching are the interventions and regulations of modern states, and the compelling reasons for this. Food is literally a vital matter for every society. Roads and pavements and parks are public spaces that depend on the state for their very existence (cf. Ripstein, 2009, ch. 8). States and only states can ensure the fair working of markets and address market failures. States, moreover, provide the legal charters that bring private companies into existence and mandate them to pursue profitability (Bakan, 2004). But regulatory regimes also set important limits on the ways in which companies can do this and, as we argued in chapter 3, can thereby empower companies to act more responsibly. No doubt, states sometimes perform these tasks badly. But that is not an argument for their not being done, but rather for their being done better. And "better," in our context, means with greater attention to children's health and well-being—something that has often lost out to powerful economic interests.

As we considered in chapter 9, schools provide a tempting and even natural forum for obesity prevention initiatives. Education about healthy lifestyles, nutritionally sound food and drink provision, and measures to combat weight-based bullying and stigma can all fit well with schools' existing responsibilities, to educate children and promote their well-being and autonomy. It may sometimes be difficult to ensure that such measures benefit disadvantaged children as much as those who are better-off, but (non-fee-paying) schools nonetheless provide a channel to reach all children in a given community, region, or even country. In addition, schools can take limited steps to increase children's awareness of the structures on which we depend for our food, and their understanding of how marketing tries to affect their choices. As such, they can help address the dangerous situation we discussed in chapter 6—one where consumers do not see, and citizens need not recognize, the complex and risky systems behind our everyday opportunities and choices. As we emphasized, none of these school-based initiatives will "solve the problem" of obesity; but they may well prove worthwhile if thoughtfully designed and evaluated.

* * *

Increasing childhood obesity rates pose difficult challenges for parents, educators, health professionals, and policymakers: How should each group respond, given their existing responsibilities and many other problems and challenges? Continuing research into the causes and effects of obesity provides a vital foundation for recommendations and policy proposals. However, responding to childhood obesity does not mean simply applying this knowledge. It also requires an awareness of the social complexity of the problem and an acknowledgment that there are many perspectives that must be brought to bear on the issues. In this book we have discussed many of the ethical and policy issues that result from this complexity. While simple solutions are unavailable, we believe that some options for action—especially at the institutional and policy levels—promise to make a contribution and are desirable for other reasons too. As we have stressed, measures to prevent childhood obesity, and to improve health more broadly, represent only some of the aims that public policy needs to take account of. Strange to tell, we may often deal better with childhood obesity by focusing on other issues besides, and by considering the wider needs of children, consumers, and citizens.

REFERENCES

Aarts, M.-J., De Vries, S. I., Van Oers, H. A., & Schuit, A. J. (2012). Outdoor play among children in relation to neighborhood characteristics: A cross-sectional neighborhood observation study. *International Journal of Behavioral Nutrition and Physical Activity, 9*, 98.

Academy of Medical Royal Colleges. (2013). Measuring up: The medical profession's prescription for the nation's obesity crisis. London. Retrieved September 18, 2013, from http://www.aomrc.org.uk/publications/statements/doc_view/9673-measuring-up.html.

Adams, J., Tyrrell, R., Adamson, A. J., & White, M. (2012). Effect of restrictions on television food advertising to children on exposure to advertisements for "less healthy" foods: Repeat cross-sectional study. *PLoS ONE, 7*(2), e31578.

Ahrens, W., Bammann, K., Siani, A., Buchecker, K., De Henauw, S., Iacoviello, L., Hebestreit, A., Krogh, V., Lissner, L., Marild, S., Molnar, D., Moreno, L. A., Pitsiladis, Y. P., Reisch, L., Tornaritis, M., Veidebaum, T., Pigeot, I., on behalf of the IDEFICS Consortium. (2011a). The IDEFICS cohort: Design, characteristics and participation in the baseline survey. *International Journal of Obesity, 35* (Supplement 1), S3–S15.

Ahrens, W., Hassel, H., Hebestreit, A., Peplies, J., Pohlabeln, H., Suling, M., & Pigeot, I. (2007). IDEFICS. Ursachen und Prävention ernährungs- und lebensstilbedingter Erkrankungen im Kindesalter. *Ernährung, 1*(7), 314–321.

Ahrens, W., Moreno, L. A., & Pigeot, I. (2011b). Childhood obesity: Prevalence worldwide—synthesis part I. In L. A. Moreno, I. Pigeot, & W. Ahrens (Eds.), *Epidemiology of obesity in children and adolescents* (pp. 219–235). New York: Springer.

Alexander, S. M., Baur, L. A., Magnusson, R., & Tobin, B. (2009). When does severe childhood obesity become a child protection issue? *The Medical Journal of Australia, 190*(3), 136–139.

Alston, J. M., Sumner, D. A., & Vosti, S. A. (2008). Farm subsidies and obesity in the United States: National evidence and international comparisons. *Food Policy, 33*(6), 470–479.

Alstott, A. L. (2004). *No exit: What parents owe their children and what society owes parents*. New York: Oxford University Press.

Anand, S. (2002). The concern for equity in health. *Journal of Epidemiology and Community Health, 56*(7), 485–487.

Anomaly, J. (2012). Is obesity a public health problem? *Public Health Ethics, 5*(3), 216–221.

Anonymous. (2003). The elephant in the room: Evolution, behavioralism, and counteradvertising in the coming war against obesity. *Harvard Law Review, 116*(4), 1161–1184.

Anonymous. (2006, September 15). Parents feed pupils through gates. *BBC News*. Retrieved December 30, 2012, from http://news.bbc.co.uk/1/hi/england/south_yorkshire/5349392.stm.

Anonymous. (2010). *Oxford Dictionary of English* (3rd ed.). Oxford: Oxford University Press.

Anonymous. (2011, July 12). Ungarisches Parlament verabschiedet "Hamburger-Steuer." Retrieved March 1, 2013, from http://www.aerzteblatt.de/nachrichten/46593/Ungarisches_Parlament_verabschiedet_Hamburger-Steuer.htm.

Anonymous. (2012, November 10). Denmark to abolish tax on high-fat food. *BBC News*. Retrieved February 25, 2013, from http://www.bbc.co.uk/news/world-europe-20280863.

Archard, D. (1990). Paternalism defined. *Analysis, 50*(1), 36–42.

Archard, D. (2003). *Children, family, and the state*. Aldershot: Ashgate.

Archard, D. (2004). *Children: Rights and childhood* (2nd ed.). New York: Routledge.

Aronson, E., Wilson, T. D., & Akert, R. M. (2012). *Social Psychology* (8th ed.). Upper Saddle River, NJ: Pearson.

Babey, S. H., Hastert, T. A., Wolstein, J., & Diamant, A. L. (2010). Income disparities in obesity trends among California adolescents. *American Journal of Public Health, 100*(11), 2149–2155.

Backett-Milburn, K. C., Wills, W. J., Gregory, S., & Lawton, J. (2006). Making sense of eating, weight and risk in the early teenage years: Views and concerns of parents in poorer socio-economic circumstances. *Social Science & Medicine, 63*(3), 624–635.

Baertlein, L., & Geller, M. (2012, September 6). Soda tax war taking shape in two California cities. Retrieved October 2, 2012, from http://www.reuters.com/article/2012/09/06/us-usa-drinks-tax-idUSBRE88507M20120906.

Bailey, T. (2012, September 20). Soda taxes will make us less free, not less fat. Retrieved October 2, 2012, from http://www.huffingtonpost.co.uk/tom-bailey/soda-taxes-will-make-us-less-free_b_1893677.html?utm_hp_ref=uk.

Bakan, J. (2004). *The corporation: The pathological pursuit of power and profit*. London: Constable.

Banack, H. R., & Kaufman, J. S. (2013). The "obesity paradox" explained. *Epidemiology, 24*(3), 461–462.

Barlow, S. E., & Expert Committee. (2007). Expert committee recommendations regarding the prevention, assessment, and treatment of child and adolescent overweight and obesity: Summary report. *Pediatrics, 120*(Supplement 4), S164–S192.

Barnhill, A. (2011). Impact and ethics of excluding sweetened beverages from the SNAP program. *American Journal of Public Health, 101*(11), 2037–2043.

Barry, C. L., Brescoll, V. L., Brownell, K. D., & Schlesinger, M. (2009). Obesity metaphors: How beliefs about the causes of obesity affect support for public policy. *The Milbank Quarterly, 87*(1), 7–47.

Barry, C. L., Gollust, S. E., & Niederdeppe, J. (2012). Are Americans ready to solve the weight of the nation? *New England Journal of Medicine, 367*(5), 389–391.

Bauer, K. W., Yang, Y. W., & Austin, S. B. (2004). "How can we stay healthy when you're throwing all of this in front of us?" Findings from focus groups and interviews in middle schools on environmental influences on nutrition and physical activity. *Health Education & Behavior, 31*(1), 34–46.

Baughcum, A. E., Chamberlin, L. A., Deeks, C. M., Powers, S. W., & Whitaker, R. C. (2000). Maternal perceptions of overweight preschool children. *Pediatrics, 106*(6), 1380–1386.

Bayer, R. (2008). Stigma and the ethics of public health: Not can we but should we. *Social Science & Medicine, 67*(3), 463–472.

Bayer, R., & Colgrove, J. (2002). Science, politics, and ideology in the campaign against environmental tobacco smoke. *American Journal of Public Health, 92*(6), 949–954.

Bayer, R., & Stuber, J. (2006). Tobacco control, stigma, and public health: Rethinking the relations. *American Journal of Public Health, 96*(1), 47–50.

Bazzocchi, A., Diano, D., & Battista, G. (2012). How fat is fat? *The Lancet, 380*(9837), e1.

Beck Research Inc., LLC. (2008). Voter preferences for closing the New York State budget gap. New York: Citizen's Committee for Children of New York, Inc. Retrieved February 25, 2013, from http://www.yaleruddcenter.org/resources/upload/docs/what/policy/SSBtaxes/NYP01112.08.pdf.

Belot, M., & James, J. (2011). Healthy school meals and educational outcomes. *Journal of Health Economics, 30*(3), 489–504.

Berg, F. M. (2005). *Underage and overweight: Our childhood obesity crisis—what every family needs to know.* Long Island City, NY: Hatherleigh Press.

Bergsma, L. J., & Carney, M. E. (2008). Effectiveness of health-promoting media literacy education: A systematic review. *Health Education Research, 23*(3), 522–542.

Bernstein, S. (2010, November 11). Restaurant group plans to fight fast-food restrictions in Los Angeles. *Los Angeles Times.* Retrieved April 4, 2013, from http://articles.latimes.com/2010/nov/11/business/la-fi-fast-food-fight-20101112.

Bertakis, K. D., & Azari, R. (2005). The impact of obesity on primary care visits. *Obesity Research, 13*(9), 1615–1623.

Bipartisan Policy Center: Nutrition and Physical Activity Initiative. (2012). Lots to lose: How America's health and obesity crisis threatens our economic future. Retrieved February 22, 2013, from http://bipartisanpolicy.org/projects/lotstolose.

Blacksher, E. (2008). Children's health inequalities: Ethical and political challenges to seeking social justice. *Hastings Center Report*, *38*(4), 28–35.

Bleich, S., & Blendon, R. J. (2011). Public opinion and obesity. In R. J. Blendon, M. Brodie, J. M. Benson, & D. E. Altman (Eds.), *American public opinion and health care*. Washington, DC: CQ Press.

Bloche, M. G. (2004). Obesity and the struggle within ourselves. *The Georgetown Law Journal*, *93*, 1335–1359.

Block, J. P., Chandra, A., McManus, K. D., & Willett, W. C. (2010). Point-of-purchase price and education intervention to reduce consumption of sugary soft drinks. *American Journal of Public Health*, *100*(8), 1427–1433.

Bocquier, A., Verger, P., Basdevant, A., Andreotti, G., Baretge, J., Villani, P., & Paraponaris, A. (2005). Overweight and obesity: Knowledge, attitudes and practices of general practitioners in France. *Obesity Research*, *13*(4), 787–795.

Booth, K. M., Pinkston, M. M., & Poston, W. S. (2005). Obesity and the built environment. *Journal of the American Dietetic Association*, *105*(5 Supplement 1), S110–S117.

Bowker, G. C., & Starr, S. L. (1999). *Sorting things out: Classification and its consequences*. Cambridge, MA: MIT Press.

Brand, J. (2007). *Television advertising to children: A review of contemporary research on the influence of television advertising directed to children*. Melbourne: Australian Communications and Media Authority. Retrieved March 7, 2013, from http://www.acma.gov.au/webwr/_assets/main/lib310132/television_advertising_to_children.pdf.

Brescoll, V. L., Kersh, R., & Brownell, K. D. (2008). Assessing the feasibility and impact of federal childhood obesity policies. *Annals of the American Academy of Political and Social Science*, *615*, 178–194.

Bridgeman, J. (1998). Case note: Criminalising the one who really cared. *Feminist Legal Studies*, *6*(2), 245–256.

Brighouse, H. (2005). Channel one, the anti-commercial principle, and the discontinuous ethos. *Educational Policy*, *19*(3), 528–549.

Brighouse, H. (2008). Education for a flourishing life. In D. Coulter & J. Wiens (Eds.), *Why do we educate? Renewing the conversation*, vol. 1 (pp. 58–71). Malden, MA: National Society for the Study of Education.

Brighouse, H. (2009). Moral and political aspects of education. In H. Siegel (Ed.), *Handbook of philosophy of education* (pp. 35–51). Oxford: Oxford University Press.

Brighouse, H., & Swift, A. (2006). Parents' rights and the value of the family. *Ethics*, *117*(1), 80–108.

Brighouse, H., & Swift, A. (2008). Putting educational equality in its place. *Education Finance and Policy*, *3*(4), 444–466.

Brighouse, H., & Swift, A. (2009). Educational equality versus educational adequacy: A critique of Anderson and Satz. *Journal of Applied Philosophy*, *26*(2), 117–128.

Brixval, C. S., Rayce, S. L. B., Rasmussen, M., Holstein, B. E., & Due, P. (2012). Overweight, body image and bullying—an epidemiological study of 11- to 15-year olds. *European Journal of Public Health, 22*(1), 126–130.

Brooks, F., & Magnusson, J. (2010). Physical activity programs in high schools. In J. O'Dea & M. Eriksen (Eds.), *Childhood obesity prevention: International research, controversies, and interventions* (pp. 380–388). New York: Oxford University Press.

Brown, H. (2010, March 15). For obese people, prejudice in plain sight. *New York Times*. Retrieved February 25, 2013, from http://www.nytimes.com/2010/03/16/health/16essa.html?_r=1.

Brownell, K. D., Farley, T., Willett, W. C., Popkin, B. M., Chaloupka, F. J., Thompson, J. W., & Ludwig, D. S. (2009). The public health and economic benefits of taxing sugar-sweetened beverages. *New England Journal of Medicine, 361*(16), 1599–1605.

Brownell, K. D., & Frieden, T. R. (2009). Ounces of prevention–The public policy case for taxes on sugared beverages. *New England Journal of Medicine, 360*(18), 1805–1808.

Brownell, K. D., Kersh, R., Ludwig, D. S., Post, R. C., Puhl, R. M., Schwartz, M. B., & Willett, W. C. (2010). Personal responsibility and obesity: A constructive approach to a controversial issue. *Health Affairs, 29*(3), 379–387.

Buchanan, D. R. (2008). Autonomy, paternalism, and justice: Ethical priorities in public health. *American Journal of Public Health, 98*(1), 15–21.

Buck, C., Pohlabeln, H., Huybrechts, I., De Bourdeaudhuij, I., Pitsiladis, Y., Reisch, L., & Pigeot, I. (2011). Development and application of a moveability index to quantify possibilities for physical activity in the build environment of children. *Health & Place, 17*(6), 1191–1201.

Buijzen, M. (2009). The effectiveness of parental communication in modifying the relation between food advertising and children's consumption behavior. *British Journal of Developmental Psychology, 27*(1), 105–121.

Buijzen, M., Rozendaal, E., Moorman, M., & Tanis, M. (2008). Parent versus child reports of parental advertising mediation: Exploring the meaning of agreement. *Journal of Broadcasting & Electronic Media, 52*(4), 509–525.

Buijzen, M., & Valkenburg, P. M. (2003). The effects of television advertising on materialism, parent-child conflict, and unhappiness: A review of research. *Journal of Applied Developmental Psychology, 24*(4), 437–456.

Buijzen, M., & Valkenburg, P. M. (2005). Parental mediation of undesired advertising effect. *Journal of Broadcasting & Electronic Media, 49*(2), 153–165.

Cain, P. (2011, June 21). Hungary for a "fat tax." *Global Post*. Retrieved February 25, 2013, from http://www.globalpost.com/dispatch/news/regions/europe/110620/hungary-fat-tax-junk-food.

Cairns, G., Angus, K., & Hastings, G. (2009). The extent, nature and effects of food promotion to children: A review of the evidence to December 2008. Geneva: World Health Organization. Retrieved May 5, 2013, from http://www.who.int/dietphysicalactivity/Evidence_Update_2009.pdf.

Callahan, D. (2013a). Obesity: Chasing an elusive epidemic. *Hastings Center Report*, 43(1), 34–40.

Callahan, D. (2013b). The author replies. *Hastings Center Report*, 43(3), 9–10.

Calle, E. E., Rodriguez, C., Walker-Thurmond, K., & Thun, M. J. (2003). Overweight, obesity, and mortality from cancer in a prospectively studied cohort of US adults. *New England Journal of Medicine*, 348(17), 1625–1638.

Cameron, N., Norgan, N., & Ellison, G. (2006). Introduction. In N. Cameron, N. Norgan, & G. Ellison (Eds.), *Childhood obesity: Contemporary issues* (pp. xix–xxviii). Boca Raton, FL: Taylor & Francis.

Campbell, D. (2010, February 28). Takeaway ban near schools to help fight child obesity. *The Guardian*. Retrieved May 25, 2013, from http://www.guardian.co.uk/society/2010/feb/28/takeaway-food-school-ban.

Campos, P. (2004). *The obesity myth*. New York: Gotham Books.

Campos, P., Saguy, A., Ernsberger, P., Oliver, E., & Gaesser, G. (2006). The epidemiology of overweight and obesity: Public health crisis or moral panic? *International Journal of Epidemiology*, 35(1), 55–60.

Caraher, M., & Cowburn, G. (2007). Taxing food: Implications for public health nutrition. *Public Health Nutrition*, 8(8), 1242–1249.

Carnell, S., Edwards, C., Croker, H., Boniface, D., & Wardle, J. (2005). Parental perceptions of overweight in 3–5 y olds. *International Journal of Obesity*, 29(4), 353–355.

Carnethon, M. R., De Chavez, P. J. D., Biggs, M. L., Lewis, C. E., Pankow, J. S., Bertoni, A. G., Golden, S. H., Liu, K., Mukamal, K. J., Campbell-Jenkins, B., & Dyer, A. R. (2012). Association of weight status with mortality in adults with incident diabetes. *Journal of the American Medical Association*, 308(6), 581–590.

Carter, O. B. J., Patterson, L. J., Donovan, R. J., Ewing, M. T., & Roberts, C. M. (2011). Children's understanding of the selling versus persuasive intent of junk food advertising: Implications for regulation. *Social Science & Medicine*, 72(6), 962–968.

Carter, R., Moodie, M., Markwick, A., Magnus, A., Vos, T., Swinburn, B., & Haby, M. M. (2009). Assessing cost-effectiveness in obesity (ACE-Obesity): An overview of the ACE approach, economic methods and cost results. *BMC Public Health*, 9(1), 419.

Carver, A., Timperio, A. F., Hesketh, K. D., & Crawford, D. A. (2012). How does perceived risk mediate associations between perceived safety and parental restriction of adolescents' physical activity in their neighborhood? *International Journal of Behavioral Nutrition and Physical Activity*, 9, 57.

Casazza, K., Fontaine, K. R., Astrup, A., Birch, L. L., Brown, A. W., Bohan Brown, M. M., Durant, N., Dutton, G., Foster, E. M., Heymsfield, S. B., McIver, K., Mehta, T., Menchemi, N., Newby, P. K., Pate, R., Rolls, B. J., Sen, B., Smith Jr, D. L., Thomas, D. M., & Allison, D. B. (2013). Myths, presumptions, and facts about obesity. *New England Journal of Medicine*, 368(5), 446–454.

Cash, S. B., & Lacanilao, R. D. (2007). Taxing food to improve health: Economic evidence and arguments. *Agricultural and Resources Economics Review*, 36(2), 174–182.

Cecchini, M., Sassi, F., Lauer, J. A., Lee, Y. V., Guajardo-Barron, V., & Chisholm, D. (2010). Tackling of unhealthy diets, physical inactivity, and obesity: Health effects and cost-effectiveness. *The Lancet, 376*(9754), 1775–1784.

Center for Science in the Public Interest. (2003). *Pestering parents: How food companies market obesity to children.* Washington, DC: Center for Science in the Public Interest. Retrieved February 14, 2013, from http://www.cspinet.org/new/200311101.html.

Centers for Disease Control and Prevention. (1999). Ten great public health achievments: United States, 1900–1999. *Morbidity and Mortality Weekly Report (MMWR), 48*(12), 241–243. Retrieved March 10, 2013, from http://www.cdc.gov/mmwr/PDF/wk/mm4812.pdf.

Chang, S.-H., Beason, T. S., Hunleth, J. M., & Colditz, G. A. (2012). A systematic review of body fat distribution and mortality in older people. *Maturitas, 72*(3), 175–191.

Chen, X., Beydoun, M. A., & Wang, Y. (2008). Is sleep duration associated with childhood obesity? A systematic review and meta-analysis. *Obesity, 16*(2), 265–274.

Cheyne, A. D., Dorfman, L., Bukofzer, E., & Harris, J. L. (2013). Marketing sugary cereals to children in the digital age: A content analysis of 17 child-targeted websites. *Journal of Health Communication: International Perspectives, 18*(5), 563–582.

Cismaru, M., & Lavack, A. M. (2007). Social marketing campaigns aimed at preventing and controlling obesity: A review and recommendations. *International Review on Public and Nonprofit Marketing, 4*(1–2), 9–30.

Claro, R. M., Levy, R. B., Popkin, B. M., & Monteiro, C. A. (2012). Sugar-sweetened beverage taxes in Brazil. *American Journal of Public Health, 102*(1), 178–183.

Clinton, H. (1996). *It takes a village: And other lessons children teach us.* New York: Simon and Shuster.

Cogan, J. C., Smith, J. P., & Maine, M. D. (2007). The risks of a quick fix: A case against mandatory body mass index reporting laws. *Eating Disorders, 16*(1), 2–13.

Cogan, J. C., Smith, J. P., & Maine, M. D. (2009). Response to critique of BMI article by Cogan, Smight and Maine. *Eating Disorders, 17*(2), 107–108.

Cohen, J. (1993). Freedom of expression. *Philosophy & Public Affairs, 22*(3), 207–263.

Cole, A., & Kmietowicz, Z. (2007). BMA rejects call for parents of obese children to be charged with neglect. *British Medical Journal, 334*(7608), 1343.

Cole, T. J., Bellizzi, M. C., Flegal, K. M., & Dietz, W. H. (2000). Establishing a standard definition for child overweight and obesity worldwide: International survey. *British Medical Journal, 320*(7244), 1240–1243.

Cole, T. J., & Rolland-Cachera, M. F. (2002). Measurement and definition. In W. Burniat, T. J. Cole, I. Lissau, & E. M. E. Poskitt (Eds.), *Child and adolescent obesity* (pp. 3–27). Cambridge: Cambridge University Press.

Commission of the European Communities. (2009). *Solidarity in health: Reducing health inequalities in the EU.* Retrieved from http://ec.europa.eu/health/ph_determinants/socio_economics/documents/com2009_en.pdf

Commission on the Social Determinants of Health. (2008). *Closing the gap in a generation: Health equity through action on the social determinants of health.* Geneva: World Health Organization.

Cook-Cottone, C., Casey, C. M., Feeley, T. H., & Baran, J. (2009). A meta-analytic review of obesity prevention in the schools: 1997–2008. *Psychology in the Schools, 46*(8), 695–719.

Couzin, J. (2005). A heavyweight battle over CDC's obesity forecasts. *Science, 308*(5723), 770–771.

Crandall, C. S. (1995). Do parents discriminate against their heavyweight daughters? *Personality and Social Psychology Bulletin, 21*(7), 724–735.

Crandall, C. S., & Reser, A. H. (2005). Attributions and weight-based prejudice. In K. D. Brownell, R. M. Puhl, M. B. Schwartz, & L. Rudd (Eds.), *Weight bias: Nature, consequences, and remedies.* New York: Guilford Press.

Croizet, J. C., & Claire, T. (1998). Extending the concept of stereotype threat to social class: The intellectual underperformance of students from low socioeconomic backgrounds. *Personality and Social Psychology Bulletin, 24*(6), 588–594.

Cuarón, A. (Director). (2006). *Children of men* [Film]. UK: Strike Entertainment/Hit and Run Productions.

Cullen, K. W., Watson, K., Zakeri, I., & Ralston, K. (2006). Exploring changes in middle-school student lunch consumption after local school food service policy modifications. *Public Health Nutrition, 9*(6), 814–820.

Curtis, J. P., Selter, J. G., Wang, Y., Rathore, S. S., Jovin, I. S., Jadbabaie, F., Kosiborod, M., Portnay, E. L., Sokol, S. I., Bader, F., & Krumholz, H. M. (2005). The obesity paradox. *Archives of Internal Medicine, 165*(1), 55–61.

Cuttini, M., & Barreto, M. L. (2010). Prevention of childhood obesity: Issues on the evaluation of interventions. *Journal of Epidemiology and Community Health, 64*(11), 939.

Daniel, L. (2012). DOD leads drive toward healthier lifestyles. Retrieved September 3, 2012, from http://www.defense.gov/news/newsarticle.aspx?id=117152.

Daniels, N. (2008). *Just health: Meeting health needs fairly.* Cambridge: Cambridge University Press.

Daniels, N., & Sabin, J. (2008). *Setting limits fairly: Learning to share resources for health* (2nd ed.). New York: Oxford University Press.

Daniels, S. R., Arnett, D. K., Eckel, R. H., Gidding, S. S., Hayman, L. L., Kumanyika, S., Robinson, T. N., Scott, B. J., St Jeor, S., & Williams, C. L. (2005). Overweight in children and adolescents: Pathophysiology, consequences, prevention, and treatment. *Circulation, 111*(15), 1999–2012.

Daníelsdóttir, S., O'Brien, K. S., & Ciao, A. (2010). Anti-fat prejudice reduction: A review of published studies. *Obesity Facts, 3*(1), 47–58.

Danish Academy of Technical Sciences. (2007). Economic nutrition policy tools—useful in the challenge to combat obesity and poor nutrition? Kongens Lyngby: Danish

Academy of Technical Sciences, ATV. Retrieved April 1, 2013, from http://www. atv.dk/uploads/1227087410economicnutrition.pdf.

Davis, M. M., Gance-Cleveland, B., Hassink, S., Johnson, R., Paradis, G., & Resnicow, K. (2007). Recommendations for prevention of childhood obesity. *Pediatrics*, *120*(Supplement 4), S229–S253.

Davison, K. K., & Birch, L. L. (2004). Predictors of fat stereotypes among 9-year-old girls and their parents. *Obesity*, *12*(1), 86–94.

Davison, K. K., & Deane, G. D. (2010). The consequence of encouraging girls to be active for weight loss. *Social Science & Medicine*, *70*(4), 518–525.

Davison, K. K., & Lawson, C. T. (2006). Do attributes in the physical environment influence children's physical activity? A review of the literature. *International Journal of Behavioral Nutrition and Physical Activity*, *3*, 19.

de Marneffe, P. (2006). Avoiding paternalism. *Philosophy & Public Affairs*, *34*(1), 68–94.

De Meester, F., Van Dyck, D., De Bourdeaudhuij, I., Deforche, B., Sallis, J. F., & Cardon, G. (2012). Active living neighborhoods: Is neighborhood walkability a key element for Belgian adolescents? *BMC Public Health*, *12*, 7.

Department of Health. (2008). *Health inequalities: Progress and next steps*. London: Department of Health.

Department of Health. (2010). *Change4Life one year on: In support of healthy weight, healthy lives*. London: Department of Health. Retrieved May 5, 2013, from http:// www.physicalactivityandnutritionwales.org.uk/Documents/740/DH_summaryof_change4lifeoneyearon.pdf.

Department of Health Public Health Research Consortium, Law, C., Power, C., Graham, H., & Merrick, D. (2007). Obesity and health inequalities. *Obesity Reviews*, *8*(s1), 19–22.

Deutsche Welle. (2005, January 22). EU considers banning junk food ads. Retrieved May 5, 2013, from http://www.dw.de/eu-considers-banning-junk-food-ads/a-1466381-1.

Dinsdale, H., Ridler, C., & Rutter, H. (2012). National child measurement programme: Changes in children's body mass index between 2006/7 and 2010/11. National Obesity Observatory. Retrieved September 18, 2012, from http://www. noo.org.uk/NCMP/National_report.

Dixey, R., Heindl, I., Loureiro, I., Pérez-Rodrigo, C., Snel, J., & Warnking, P. (1999). *Healthy eating for young people in Europe: A school-based nutrition education guide*. Copenhagen: International Planning Committee of the European Network of Health Promoting Schools.

Doak, C., Heitmann, B. L., Summerbell, C. D., & Lissner, L. (2009). Prevention of childhood obesity—what type of evidence should we consider relevant? *Obesity Reviews*, *10*(3), 350–356.

Doak, C., Visscher, T., Renders, C., & Seidell, J. (2006). The prevention of overweight and obesity in children and adolescents: A review of interventions and programmes. *Obesity Reviews*, *7*(1), 111–136.

Dole, B. (1996). Address accepting the presidential nomination at the Republican National Convention, San Diego, August 15. Retrieved March 5, 2013, from http://www.pbs.org/newshour/convention96/floor_speeches/bob_dole.html.

Doyle, C. (2003, November 21). Defusing the child obesity time bomb. *Daily Telegraph.* Retrieved February 22, 2013, from http://www.telegraph.co.uk/health/3303555/Defusing-the-child-obesity-time-bomb.html.

Drewnowski, A., & Darmon, N. (2005). The economics of obesity: Dietary energy density and energy cost. *American Journal of Clinical Nutrition, 82* (1 Supplement), 265–273.

Due, P., Damsgaard, M., Rasmussen, M., Holstein, B., Wardle, J., Merlo, J., Currie, C., Ahluwalia, N., Sørensen, T., & Lynch, J., and the HSBC obesity writing group (2009). Socioeconomic position, macroeconomic environment and overweight among adolescents in 35 countries. *International Journal of Obesity, 33*(10), 1084–1093.

Dunton, G., Kaplan, J., Wolch, J., Jerrett, M., & Reynolds, K. (2009). Physical environmental correlates of childhood obesity: A systematic review. *Obesity Reviews, 10*(4), 393–402.

Dworkin, G. (2010). Paternalism. In E. N. Zalta (Ed.), *The Stanford Encyclopedia of Philosophy* (Summer 2010 ed.). Retrieved February 25, 2013, from http://plato.stanford.edu/archives/sum2010/entries/paternalism.

Ebbeling, C. B., & Ludwig, D. S. (2008). Tracking pediatric obesity: An index of uncertainty? *Journal of the American Medical Association, 299*(20), 2442–2443.

Edmunds, L. (2005). Parents' perceptions of health professionals' responses when seeking help for their overweight children. *Family Practice, 22*(3), 287–292.

Eisenberg, M. E., Neumark-Sztainer, D., Haines, J., & Wall, M. (2006). Weight-teasing and emotional well-being in adolescents: Longitudinal findings from Project EAT. *Journal of Adolescent Health, 38*(6), 675–683.

Eisenberg, M. E., Neumark-Sztainer, D., & Story, M. (2003). Associations of weight-based teasing and emotional well-being among adolescents. *Archives of Pediatrics and Adolescent Medicine, 157*(8), 733–738.

Elinder, L. S. (2005). Obesity, hunger, and agriculture: The damaging role of subsidies. *British Medical Journal, 331*(7528), 1333–1336.

Engster, D. (2010). The place of parenting within a liberal theory of justice. *Social Theory & Practice, 36*(2), 233–262.

Epstein, L. H., Dearing, K. K., Paluch, R. A., Roemmich, J. N., & Cho, D. (2007). Price and maternal obesity influence purchasing of low- and high-energy-dense foods. *American Journal of Clinical Nutrition, 86*(4), 914–922.

Epstein, L. H., Dearing, K. K., Roba, L. G., & Finkelstein, E. (2010). The influence of taxes and subsidies on energy purchased in an experimental purchasing study. *Psychological Science, 21*(3), 406–414.

Epstein, L. H., Roemmich, J. N., Robinson, J. L., Paluch, R. A., Winiewicz, D. D., Fuerch, J. H., & Robinson, T. N. (2008). A randomized trial of the effects of reducing television viewing and computer use on body mass index in young children. *Archives of Pediatrics and Adolescent Medicine, 162*(3), 239–245.

Epstein, R. A. (2003). Let the shoemaker stick to his last: A defense of the "old" public health. *Perspectives in Biology and Medicine, 46*(3), S138–S159.

Erickson, S. J., Robinson, T. N., Haydel, K. F., & Killen, J. D. (2000). Are overweight children unhappy? Body mass index, depressive symptoms, and overweight concerns in elementary school children. *Archives of Pediatrics & Adolescent Medicine, 154*(9), 931–935.

European Commission: Directorate-General for Agriculture and Rural Development. (2012). School fruit scheme: Overview. Retrieved August 31, 2012, from http://ec.europa.eu/agriculture/sfs/index_en.html.

Evans, B., & Colls, R. (2011). Doing more good than harm? The absent presence of children's bodies in (anti-)obesity policy. In E. Rich, L. F. Monahan, & L. Aphramor (Eds.), *Debating obesity: Critical perspectives* (pp. 115–138). Houndmills, UK: Palgrave Macmillan.

Evans, C. E. L., Greenwood, D. C., Thomas, J. D., & Cade, J. E. (2010). A cross-sectional survey of children's packed lunches in the UK: Food- and nutrient-based results. *Journal of Epidemiology and Community Health, 64*(11), 977–983.

Evans, W. D. (2006). How social marketing works in health care. *British Medical Journal, 332*(7551), 1207–1210.

Faith, M. S., Leone, M. A., Ayers, T. S., Heo, M., & Pietrobelli, A. (2002). Weight criticism during physical activity, coping skills, and reported physical activity in children. *Pediatrics, 110*(2), e23.

Farley, T. A., Meriwether, R. A., Baker, E. T., Watkins, L. T., Johnson, C. C., & Webber, L. S. (2007). Safe play spaces to promote physical activity in inner-city children: Results from a pilot study of an environmental intervention. *American Journal of Public Health, 97*(9), 1625–1631.

Ferdinand, A. O., Sen, B., Rahurkar, S., Engler, S., & Menachemi, N. (2012). The relationship between built environments and physical activity: A systematic review. *American Journal of Public Health, 102*(10), e7-e13

Ferrante, J. M., Chen, P. H., Crabtree, B. F., & Wartenberg, D. (2007). Cancer screening in women: Body mass index and adherence to physician recommendations. *American Journal of Preventive Medicine, 32*(6), 525–531.

Finkelstein, E., French, S., Variyam, J. N., & Haines, P. S. (2004). Pros and cons of proposed interventions to promote healthy eating. *American Journal of Preventive Medicine, 27*(3 Supplement), 163–171.

Finkelstein, E. A., & Zuckerman, L. (2008). *The fattening of America: How the economy makes us fat, if it matters, and what to do about it.* Hoboken, NJ: John Wiley.

Finucane, M. M., Stevens, G. A., Cowan, M. J., Danaei, G., Lin, J. K., Paciorek, C. J., Singh, G. M., Gutierrez, H. R., Lu, Y., Bahalim, A. N. Farzadfar, F., Riley, L.M., & Ezzati, M., on behalf of the Global Burden of Metabolic Risk Factors of Chronic Diseases Collaborating Group (Body Mass Index). (2011). National, regional, and global trends in body-mass index since 1980: Systematic analysis of health examination surveys and epidemiological studies with 960 country-years and 9.1 million participants. *The Lancet, 377*(9765), 557–567.

Fischler, C. (2011). Commensality, society and culture. *Social Science Information, 50*(3–4), 528–548.

Flegal, K. M. (1993). Defining obesity in children and adolescents: Epidemiologic approaches. *Critical Reviews in Food Science and Nutrition, 33*(4–5), 307–312.

Flegal, K. M. (2006). Commentary: The epidemic of obesity—what's in a name? *International Journal of Epidemiology, 35*(1), 72–74.

Flegal, K. M. (2012). The conundrum of smoking cessation and weight gain. *Preventive Medicine, 54*(3–4), 193–194.

Flegal, K. M., Carroll, M. D., Kit, B. K., & Ogden, C. L. (2012). Prevalence of obesity and trends in the distribution of body mass index among US adults, 1999–2010. *Journal of the American Medical Association, 307*(5), 491–497.

Flegal, K. M., Tabak, C. J., & Ogden, C. L. (2006). Overweight in children: Definitions and interpretation. *Health Education Research, 21*(6), 755–760.

Flodmark, C. E., Marcus, C., & Britton, M. (2006). Interventions to prevent obesity in children and adolescents: A systematic literature review. *International Journal of Obesity, 30*(4), 579–589.

Food and Drink Federation. (n.d.). FDF's response to Ofcom consultation: "Television advertising of food and drink products to children." Retrieved March 12, 2011, from http://stakeholders.ofcom.org.uk/binaries/consultations/foodads_new/responses/fdf.pdf.

Food Ethics Council. (2005). *Getting personal: Shifting responsibilities for dietary health.* Brighton: Food Ethics Council. Retrieved May 8, 2013, from http://www.foodethicscouncil.org/node/110.

Foresight. (2007). *Tackling obesities: Future choices. Project report* (2nd ed.). London: Department for Business, Innovation & Skills.

Fox, C. L., & Farrow, C. V. (2009). Global and physical self-esteem and body dissatisfaction as mediators of the relationship between weight status and being a victim of bullying. *Journal of Adolescence, 32*(5), 1287–1301.

Fox, M. K., Gordon, A., Nogales, R., & Wilson, A. (2009). Availability and consumption of competitive foods in US public schools. *Journal of the American Dietetic Association, 109*(2 Supplement), S57–S66.

Freedman, D. S., Dietz, W. H., Srinivasan, S. R., & Berenson, G. S. (2009). Risk factors and adult body mass index among overweight children: The Bogalusa Heart Study. *Pediatrics, 123*(3), 750–757.

Freedman, D. S., Khan, L. K., Serdula, M. K., Dietz, W. H., Srinivasan, S. R., & Berenson, G. S. (2005). The relation of childhood BMI to adult adiposity: The Bogalusa Heart Study. *Pediatrics, 115*(1), 22–27.

French, S. A., Jeffery, R. W., Story, M., Breitlow, K. K., Baxter, J. S., Hannan, P., & Snyder, M. P. (2001). Pricing and promotion effects on low-fat vending snack purchases: The CHIPS study. *American Journal of Public Health, 91*(1), 112–117.

Friedman, J. (2004). Modern science versus the stigma of obesity. *Nature Medicine*, *10*(6), 563–569.

Friedman, R. R., & Brownell, K. D. (2012). Sugar-sweetened beverage taxes: An updated policy brief. New Haven, CT: Yale Rudd Center for Food Policy and Obesity. Retrieved February 25, 2013, from http://www.yaleruddcenter.org/resources/upload/docs/what/reports/Rudd_Policy_Brief_Sugar_Sweetened_Beverage_Taxes.pdf.

Friel, S., Chopra, M., & Satcher, D. (2007). Unequal weight: Equity oriented policy responses to the global obesity epidemic. *British Medical Journal*, *335*(7632), 1241–1243.

Friel, S., Kelleher, C., Campbell, P., & Nolan, G. (1999). Evaluation of the nutrition education at primary school (NEAPS) programme. *Public Health Nutrition*, *2*(4), 549–555.

Fuemmeler, B. F., Baffi, C., Mâsse, L. C., Atienza, A. A., & Evans, W. D. (2007). Employer and healthcare policy interventions aimed at adult obesity. *American Journal of Preventive Medicine*, *32*(1), 44–51.

Furedi, F. (2002). *Paranoid parenting: Why ignoring the experts may be best for your child*. Chicago, IL: Chicago Review Press.

Gable, S., Krull, J., & Srikanta, A. (2008). Childhood overweight and academic achievement. In H. Fitzgerald & V. Mousouli (Eds.), *Obesity in childhood and adolescence (Volume 2: Understanding Development and Prevention)* (pp. 49–72). Westport, CT: Praeger.

Gard, M. (2011a). *The end of the obesity epidemic*. London: Routledge.

Gard, M. (2011b). Truth, belief and the cultural politics of obesity scholarship and public health policy. Critical Public Health, 21(1), 37–48.

Gibbs, W. W. (2005). Obesity: An overblown epidemic? *Scientific American*, *292*(6), 70–77.

Gibson, L., Byrne, S., Davis, E., Blair, E., Jacoby, P., & Zubrick, S. (2007). The role of family and maternal factors in childhood obesity. *Medical Journal of Australia*, *186*(11), 591–595.

Giskes, K., Van Lenthe, F. J., Brug, J., Mackenbach, J., & Turrell, G. (2007). Socioeconomic inequalities in food purchasing: The contribution of respondent-perceived and actual (objectively measured) price and availability of foods. *Preventive Medicine*, *45*(1), 41–48.

Goffman, E. (1963). *Stigma: Notes on the management of spoiled identity*. Englewood Cliffs, NJ: Penguin.

Goldschmidt, A. B., Hilbert, A., Manwaring, J. L., Wilfley, D. E., Pike, K. M., Fairburn, C. G., Dohm, F. A., & Striegel-Moore, R. H. (2010). The significance of overvaluation of shape and weight in binge eating disorder. *Behaviour Research and Therapy*, *48*(3), 187–193.

Gordon, R., McDermott, L., Stead, M., & Angus, K. (2006). The effectiveness of social marketing interventions for health improvement: What's the evidence? *Public Health*, *120*(12), 1133–1139.

Goris, J. M., Petersen, S., Stamatakis, E., & Veerman, J. L. (2010). Television food advertising and the prevalence of childhood overweight and obesity: A multicountry comparison. *Public Health Nutrition*, *13*(7), 1003–1012.

Gortmaker, S. L., Dietz Jr., W. H., Sobol, A. M., & Wehler, C. A. (1987). Increasing pediatric obesity in the United States. *American Journal of Diseases in Children*, *141*(5), 535–540.

Grier, S., & Bryant, C. A. (2005). Social marketing in public health. *Public Health*, *26*(1), 319–339.

Grün, F. (2010). Obesogens. *Current Opinion in Endocrinology, Diabetes & Obesity*, *17*(5), 453–459.

Grün, F., & Blumberg, B. (2009). Minireview: The case for obesogens. *Molecular Endocrinology*, *23*(8), 1127–1134.

Grynbaum, M. M. (2012). Will soda restrictions help New York win the war on obesity? *British Medical Journal*, *345*, e6768.

Guthman, J. (2011). *Weighing in: Obesity, food justice, and the limits of capitalism.* Berkley: University of California Press.

Gutmann, A. (1980). Children, paternalism, and education: A liberal argument. *Philosophy & Public Affairs*, *9*(4), 338–358.

Gwozdz, W., & Reisch, L. A., on behalf of the IDEFICS consortium (2011). Instruments for analyzing the influence of advertising on children's food choices. *International Journal of Obesity*, *35*, S137–S143.

Haerens, L., De Bourdeaudhuij, I., Barba, G., Eiben, G., Fernandez, J., Hebestreit, A., Kovács, É., Lasn, H., Regber, S., & Shiakou, M., on behalf of the IDEFICS consortium (2009). Developing the IDEFICS community-based intervention program to enhance eating behaviors in 2- to 8-year-old children: Findings from focus groups with children and parents. *Health Education Research*, *24*(3), 381–393.

Haines, J. (2010). Weight-related teasing and anti-teasing initiatives in schools. In J. O'Dea & M. Eriksen (Eds.), *Childhood obesity prevention: International research, controversies, and interventions* (pp. 363–379). New York: Oxford University Press.

Haines, J., Neumark-Sztainer, D., Perry, C., Hannan, P., & Levine, M. (2006). VIK (Very Important Kids): A school-based program designed to reduce teasing and unhealthy weight-control behaviors. *Health Education Research*, *21*(6), 884–895.

Haji, I., & Cuypers, S. E. (2008). Authenticity sensitive preferentialism and educating for well-being and autonomy. *Journal of Philosophy of Education*, *42*(1), 85–106.

Hammer, L. D. (2010). Childhood obesity: Treatment or prevention? In J. A. O'Dea & M. Erisken (Eds.), *Childhood obesity prevention: International research, controversies, and interventions* (pp. 195–202). New York: Oxford University Press.

Hand, M. (2002). Religious upbringing reconsidered. *Journal of Philosophy of Education*, *36*(4), 545–557.

Hand, M. (2006). Against autonomy as an educational aim. *Oxford Review of Education*, *32*(4), 535–550.

Handsley, E., Mehta, K., Coveney, J., & Nehmy, C. (2009). Regulatory axes on food advertising to children on television. *Australia and New Zealand Health Policy*, 6, 1.

Hanks, A. S., Just, D. R., Smith, L. E., & Wansink, B. (2012). Healthy convenience: Nudging students toward healthier choices in the lunchroom. *Journal of Public Health*, *34*(3), 370–376.

Hardus, P. M., van Vuuren, C. L., Crawford, D., & Worsley, A. (2003). Public perceptions of the causes and prevention of obesity among primary school children. *International Journal of Obesity*, *27*(12), 1465–1471.

Harlan, W. R., Landis, J. R., Flegal, K. M., Davis, C. S., & Miller, M. E. (1988). Secular trends in body mass in the United States, 1960–1980. *American Journal of Epidemiology*, *128*(5), 1065–1074.

Harriger, J., Calogero, R., Witherington, D., & Smith, J. (2010). Body size stereotyping and internalization of the thin ideal in preschool girls. *Sex Roles*, *63*(9), 609–620.

Harris, J. L., Bargh, J. A., & Brownell, K. D. (2009a). Priming effects of television food advertising on eating behavior. *Health Psychology*, *28*(4), 404–413.

Harris, J. L., Brownell, K., & Bargh, J. (2009b). The food marketing defense model: Integrating psychological research to protect youth and inform public policy. *Social Issues and Policy Review*, *3*(1), 211–271.

Harris, J. L., Pomeranz, J. L., Lobstein, T., & Brownell, K. D. (2009c). A crisis in the marketplace: How food marketing contributes to childhood obesity and what can be done. *Annual Review of Public Health*, *30*(1), 211–225.

Harris, J. L., Milici, F. F., Sarda, V., & Schwartz, M. B. (2012). *Food marketing to children and adolescents: What do parents think?* New Haven, CT: Yale Rudd Center for Food Policy and Obesity. Retrieved May 5, 2013, from http://www.yaleruddcenter.org/resources/upload/docs/what/reports/Rudd_Report_Parents_Survey_Food_Marketing_2012.pdf.

Haskins, R., Paxson, C., & Donahue, E. (2006). Fighting obesity in the public schools. *Future of children policy brief.* Retrieved May 3, 2013, from http://futureofchildren.org/futureofchildren/publications/docs/16_01_PolicyBrief.pdf.

Hastings, G., & McDermott, L. (2006). Putting social marketing into practice. *British Medical Journal*, *332*(7551), 1210–1212.

Hastings, G., McDermott, L., Angus, K., Stead, M., & Thomson, S. (2006). The extent, nature and effects of food promotion to children: A review of the evidence. Geneva: World Health Organization. Retrieved May 5, 2013, from http://www.who.int/dietphysicalactivity/publications/Hastings_paper_marketing.pdf.

Hastings, G., Stead, M., & McDermott, L. (2004). From the billboard to the school canteen: How food promotion influences children. *Education Review*, *17*(2), 17–23.

Hatch, E. E., Nelson, J. W., Stahlhut, R. W., & Webster, T. F. (2010). Association of endocrine disruptors and obesity: Perspectives from epidemiological studies. *International Journal of Andrology*, *33*(2), 324–332.

Hausman, D., & Welch, B. (2010). Debate: To nudge or not to nudge. *Journal of Political Philosophy*, *18*(1), 123–136.

Hawkes, C. (2005). Self-regulation of food advertising: What it can, could and cannot do to discourage unhealthy eating habits among children. *Nutrition Bulletin, 30*(4), 374–382.

Hawkes, N. (2008). National obesity strategy: What's the big idea? *British Medical Journal, 337,* 1204.

Head, B. W. (2008). Three lenses of evidence-based policy. *Australian Journal of Public Administration, 67*(1), 1–11.

Hebden, L. A., King, L., Grunseit, A., Kelly, B., & Chapman, K. (2011). Advertising of fast food to children on Australian television: The impact of industry self-regulation. *The Medical Journal of Australia, 195*(1), 20–24.

Hebl, M. R., & Xu, J. (2001). Weighing the care: Physicians' reactions to the size of a patient. *International Journal of Obesity, 25*(8), 1246–1252.

Herman, K. M., Craig, C. L., Gauvin, L., & Katzmarzyk, P. T. (2009). Tracking of obesity and physical activity from childhood to adulthood: The Physical Activity Longitudinal Study. *International Journal of Pediatric Obesity, 4*(4), 281–288.

Herndon, A. M. (2010). Mommy made me do it: Mothering fat children in the midst of the obesity epidemic. *Food Culture & Society, 13*(3), 331–349.

Herrick, C. (2007). Risky bodies: Public health, social marketing and the governance of obesity. *Geoforum, 38*(1), 90–102.

Hesketh, K., Wake, M., Waters, E., Carlin, J., & Crawford, D. (2003). Stability of body mass index in Australian children: A prospective cohort study across the middle childhood years. *Public Health Nutrition, 7*(2), 303–309.

Hillier, F., Pedley, C., & Summerbell, C. (2011). Evidence base for primary prevention of obesity in children and adolescents. *Bundesgesundheitsblatt-Gesundheitsforschung-Gesundheitsschutz, 54*(3), 259–264.

Himes, J. H., & Dietz, W. H. (1994). Guidelines for overweight in adolescent preventive services: Recommendations from an expert committee. *The American Journal of Clinical Nutrition, 59*(2), 307–316.

Hindin, T. J., Contento, I. R., & Gussow, J. D. (2004). A media literacy nutrition education curriculum for head start parents about the effects of television advertising on their children's food requests. *Journal of the American Dietetic Association, 104*(2), 192–198.

Holm, S. (2007). Obesity interventions and ethics. *Obesity Reviews, 8*(Supplement 1), 207–210.

Holm, S. (2008). Parental responsibility and obesity in children. *Public Health Ethics, 1*(1), 21–29.

Horne, M. (2010, March 21). Schools take the biscuit and the cake. *The Sunday Times,* 10.

Hossain, P., Kawar, B., & El Nahas, M. (2007). Obesity and diabetes in the developing world—a growing challenge. *New England Journal of Medicine, 356*(3), 213–215.

Hubbard, V. S. (2000). Defining overweight and obesity: What are the issues? *American Journal of Clinical Nutrition, 72*(5), 1067–1068.

Hughes, C. C., Sherman, S. N., & Whitaker, R. C. (2010). How low-income mothers with overweight preschool children make sense of obesity. *Qualitative Health Research*, 20(4), 465–478.

Huhman, M. E., Potter, L. D., Nolin, M. J., Piesse, A., Judkins, D. R., Banspach, S. W., & Wong, F. L. (2010). The influence of the verb campaign on children's physical activity in 2002 to 2006. *American Journal of Public Health*, 100(4), 638–645.

Hunsberger, M., Lanfer, A., Reeske, A., Veidebaum, T., Russo, P., Hadjigeorgiou, C., Moreno, L. A., Molnar, D., De Henauw, S., Lissner, L., & Eibern, G. (2012). Infant feeding practices and prevalence of obesity in eight European countries—the IDEFICS study. *Public Health Nutrition*, 16(2), 219–227.

Inglis, V., Ball, K., & Crawford, D. (2005). Why do women of low socioeconomic status have poorer dietary behaviours than women of higher socioeconomic status? A qualitative exploration. *Appetite*, 45(3), 334–343.

Iobst, E. A., Ritchey, P. N., Nabors, L. A., Stutz, R., Ghee, K., & Smith, D. T. (2009). Children's acceptance of a peer who is overweight: Relations among gender, age and blame for weight status. *International Journal of Obesity*, 33(7), 736–742.

Irving, L. (2000). Promoting size acceptance in elementary school children: The EDAP Puppet Program. *Eating Disorders*, 8(3), 221–232.

Jain, A., Sherman, S. N., Chamberlin, L. A., Carter, Y., Powers, S. W., & Whitaker, R. C. (2001). Why don't low-income mothers worry about their preschoolers being overweight? *Pediatrics*, 107(5), 1138–1146.

James, P. D. (1992). *Children of men*. London: Faber & Faber.

Jensen, J. D., & Smed, S. (2007). Cost-effective design of economic instruments in nutrition policy. *International Journal of Behavioral Nutrition and Physical Activity*, 4, 10.

Jensen, J. D., & Smed, S. (2012). The Danish tax on saturated fat: Short run effects on consumption and consumer prices of fats. FOI Working Paper. Copenhagen: Institute of Food and Resource Economics, University of Copenhagen. Retrieved April 1, 2013, from http://okonomi.foi.dk/workingpapers/WPpdf/WP2012/WP_2012_14_Danish_fat_tax.pdf.

Jiang, J., Xia, X., Greiner, T., Wu, G., Lian, G., & Rosenqvist, U. (2007). The effects of a 3-year obesity intervention in schoolchildren in Beijing. *Child: Care, Health & Development*, 33(5), 641–646.

Johnson, F., Pratt, M., & Wardle, J. (2011). Socio-economic status and obesity in childhood. In L. Moreno, I. Pigeot, & W. Ahrens (Eds.), *Epidemiology of obesity in children and adolescents: Prevalence and etiology* (pp. 377–390). New York: Springer.

Jones, M. M., & Bayer, R. (2007). Paternalism and its discontents: Motorcycle helmet laws, libertarian values, and public health. *American Journal of Public Health*, 97(2), 208–217.

Jones, S. C., Mannino, N., & Green, J. (2006). "Like me, want me, buy me, eat me": Relationship-building marketing communications in children's magazines. *Public Health Nutrition*, 13(12), 2111–2118.

Jutel, A. (2006). The emergence of overweight as a disease entity: Measuring up normality. *Social Science & Medicine*, *63*(9), 2268–2276.

Jutel, A. (2009). Sociology of diagnosis: A preliminary review. *Sociology of Health & Illness*, *31*(2), 278–299.

Kaiser Family Foundation. (2003). Key facts—media literacy. Retrieved March 13, 2011, from http://www.kff.org/entmedia/upload/Key-Facts-Media-Literacy.pdf.

Katz, D. L. (2012). Childhood obesity and eating disorders: Horns of a dilemma or faces of a coin? *Childhood Obesity*, *8*(5), 415–416.

Kawachi, I., Subramanian, S. V., & Almeida-Filho, N. (2002). A glossary for health inequalities. *Journal of Epidemiology and Community Health*, *56*(9), 647–652.

Keery, H., Boutelle, K., van den Berg, P., & Thompson, J. K. (2005). The impact of appearance-related teasing by family members. *Journal of Adolescent Health*, *37*(2), 120–127.

Kelly, B., Halford, J. C., Boyland, E. J., Chapman, K., Bautista-Castaño, I., Berg, C., Caroli, M., Cook, B., Coutinho, J. G., Effertz, T., Grammatikaki, E., Keller, K., Leung, R., Manios, Y., Monteiro, R., Redley, C., Prell, H., Raine, K., Recine, E., Serra-Majem, L., Singh, S., & Summerbell, C. (2010). Television food advertising to children: A global perspective. *American Journal of Public Health*, *100*(9), 1730–1736.

Kent, M. P., Dubois, L., & Wanless, A. (2011). Internet marketing to children on food/beverage websites in two different policy environments. *Obesity Reviews*, *12*(Supplement 1), 22.

Kessler, D. A. (2009). *The end of overeating: Taking control of the insatiable American appetite*. New York: Rodale Books.

Kim, S. H., & Willis, L. A. (2007). Talking about obesity: News framing of who is responsible for causing and fixing the problem. *Journal of Health Communication*, *12*(4), 359–376.

Kinge, J. M., & Morris, S. (2010). Socioeconomic variation in the impact of obesity on health related quality of life. *Social Science & Medicine*, *71*(10), 1864–1871.

Kinra, S., Nelder, R. P., & Lewendon, G. J. (2000). Deprivation and childhood obesity: A cross sectional study of 20,973 children in Plymouth, United Kingdom. *Journal of Epidemiology and Community Health*, *54*(6), 456–460.

Kirchengast, S., & Schober, E. (2006). To be an immigrant: A risk factor for developing overweight and obesity during childhood and adolescence? *Journal of Biosocial Science*, *38*(6), 695–705.

Kirk, S. F., Penney, T. L., & McHugh, T. L. F. (2010). Characterizing the obesogenic environment: The state of the evidence with directions for future research. *Obesity Reviews*, *11*(2), 109–117.

Kluck, A. S. (2010). Family influence on disordered eating: The role of body image dissatisfaction. *Body Image*, *7*(1), 8–14.

Kotler, P., Lee, N. R., & Lee, N. (2008). *Social marketing: Influencing behaviors for good* (3rd ed.). Los Angeles, CA: Sage.

Kraig, K. A., & Keel, P. K. (2001). Weight-based stigmatization in children. *International Journal of Obesity, 25*(11), 1661–1666.

Krebs, J., & Schmidt, H. (2009). Ethics and public health: The ethics of intervention choices. In A. Killoran & M. Kelly (Eds.), *Evidence-based public health, effectiveness and efficiency* (pp. 169–182). Oxford: Oxford University Press.

Krukowski, R. A., West, D. S., Perez, A. P., Bursac, Z., Phillips, M. M., & Raczynski, J. M. (2009). Overweight children, weight-based teasing and academic performance. *International Journal of Pediatric Obesity, 4*(4), 274–280.

Kuchler, F., Tegene, A., & Harris, J. M. (2004). Taxing snack foods: What to expect for diet and tax revenues. *Agriculture Information Bulletin, 747*–08, 1–11.

Kuczmarski, R. J., & Flegal, K. M. (2000). Criteria for definition of overweight in transition: Background and recommendations for the United States. *American Journal of Clinical Nutrition, 72*(5), 1074–1081.

Kuipers, Y. (2010). Focusing on obesity through a health equity lens. Retrieved August 11, 2010, from http://www.equitychannel.net/uploads/REPORT—Focusing on Obesity through a Health Health Equity Lens—Edition 2.pdf.

Kumanyika, S., & Grier, S. (2006). Targeting interventions for ethnic minority and low-income populations. *The Future of Children, 16*(1), 187–207.

Kunešová, M., Vignerová, J., Pařízková, J., Procházka, B., Braunerová, R., Riedlová, J., Zamrazilová, H., Hill, M., Bláha, P., & Šteflová, A. (2011). Long-term changes in prevalence of overweight and obesity in Czech 7-year-old children: Evaluation of different cut-off criteria of childhood obesity. *Obesity Reviews, 12*(7), 483–491.

La Caze, A., & Colyvan, M. (2006). Evidence-based policy: Promises and challenges. Retrieved March 6, 2013, from http://www.colyvan.com/papers/ebp.pdf.

Labree, L. J., van de Mheen, H., Rutten, F. F., & Foets, M. (2011). Differences in overweight and obesity among children from migrant and native origin: A systematic review of the European literature. *Obesity Reviews, 12*(5), e535–e547.

Lamerz, A., Kuepper-Nybelen, J., Wehle, C., Bruning, N., Trost-Brinkhues, G., Brenner, H., Hebebrand, J., & Herpertz-Dahlmann, B. (2005). Social class, parental education, and obesity prevalence in a study of six-year-old children in Germany. *International Journal of Obesity, 29*(4), 373–380.

Lang, T., Barling, D., & Caraher, M. (2009). *Food policy: Integrating health, environment and society.* New York: Oxford University Press.

Lang, T., & Rayner, G. (2005). Obesity: A growing issue for European policy? *Journal of European Social Policy, 15*(4), 301–327.

Lang, T., & Rayner, G. (2007). Overcoming policy cacophony on obesity: An ecological public health framework for policymakers. *Obesity Reviews, 8*(Supplement 1), 165–181.

Langnäse, K., Asbeck, I., Mast, M., & Müller, M. J. (2004). The influence of socio-economic status on the long-term effect of family-based obesity treatment intervention in prepubertal overweight children. *Health Education, 104*(6), 336–343.

Lareau, A. (2011). *Unequal childhoods: Class, race, and family life* (2nd ed. with an update a decade later). Berkeley: University of California Press.

Larson, N. I., Neumark-Sztainer, D., & Story, M. (2009). Weight control behaviors and dietary intake among adolescents and young adults: Longitudinal findings from Project EAT. *Journal of the American Dietetic Association, 109*(11), 1869–1877.

Lasserre, A. M., Chiolero, A., Cachat, F., Paccaud, F., & Bovet, P. (2007). Overweight in Swiss children and associations with children's and parents' characteristics. *Obesity, 15*(12), 2912–2919.

Latner, J. D., & Schwartz, M. B. (2005). Weight bias in a child's world. In K. D. Brownell, R. M. Puhl, M. B. Schwartz, & L. Rudd (Eds.), *Weight bias: Nature, consequences, and remedies* (pp. 54–67). New York: Guildford Press.

Latner, J. D., & Stunkard, A. J. (2003). Getting worse: The stigmatization of obese children. *Obesity, 11*(3), 452–456.

Latner, J. D., Wilson, G. T., Jackson, M. L., & Stunkard, A. J. (2009). Greater history of weight-related stigmatizing experience is associated with greater weight loss in obesity treatment. *Journal of Health Psychology, 14*(2), 190–199.

Lawrence, F. (2008). *Eat your heart out: Why the food business is bad for the planet and your health*. London: Penguin.

Le Grand, J., & Srivastava, D. (2009). *Incentives for prevention*. London: Health England.

Lee, M.-J., Popkin, B.M., & Kim, S. (2002). The unique aspects of the nutrition transition in South Korea: The retention of healthful elements in their traditional diet. *Public Health Nutrition, 5*(1a), 197–203.

Leicester, A., & Windmeijer, F. (2004). The "fat tax": Economic incentives to reduce obesity (Briefing Note No. 49). London: The Institute for Fiscal Studies. Retrieved February 25, 2013, from http:///www.ifs.org.uk/bns/bn49.pdf.

Lemmen, R. (2005). Media education in European schools. Retrieved March 12, 2011, from http://www.mediaed.org.uk/content/view/84/115/.

Leonard, A. (2010). *The story of stuff: How our obsession with stuff is trashing the planet, our communities, and our health and a vision for change*. New York: Free Press.

Leonhardt, D. (2009, May 19). Sodas a tempting tax target. *New York Times*. Retrieved October 24, 2012, from http://www.nytimes.com/2009/05/20/business/economy/201eonhardt.html.

Levi, J., Segal, L., Lang, A., & Rayburn, J. (2012). F as in fat: How obesity threatens America's future—2012. Washington DC: Trust for America's Health / Robert Wood Johnson Foundation. Retrieved March 6, 2013, from http://healthamericans.org/report/100/.

Lewis, S., Thomas, S. L., Hyde, J., Castle, D., Blood, R., & Komesaroff, P. A. (2010). "I don't eat a hamburger and large chips every day!" A qualitative study of the impact of public health messages about obesity on obese adults. *BMC Public Health, 10*, 309.

Libbey, H. P., Story, M. T., Neumark-Sztainer, D. R., & Boutelle, K. N. (2008). Teasing, disordered eating behaviors, and psychological morbidities among overweight adolescents. *Obesity, 16*(Supplement 2), S24–S29.

Lichtenstein, A. H., & Ludwig, D. S. (2010). Bringing back home economics education. *Journal of the American Medical Association, 303*(18), 1857–1858.

Lien, N., Henriksen, H. B., Nymoen, L. L., Wind, M., & Klepp, K.-I. (2010). Availability of data assessing the prevalence and trends of overweight and obesity among European adolescents. *Public Health, 13*(10A), 1680–1687.

Link, B. G., & Phelan, J. (2006). Stigma and its public health implications. *The Lancet, 367*(9509), 528–529.

Livingstone, S., & Helsper, E. J. (2006). Does advertising literacy mediate the effects of advertising on children? A critical examination of two linked research literatures in relation to obesity and food choice. *Journal of Communication, 56*(3), 560–584.

Lobstein, T. (2005). Commentary: Obesity—public health crisis, moral panic or a human rights issue? *International Journal of Epidemiology, 35*(1), 74–76.

Lobstein, T. (2009). Letter to the editor: Marketing of unhealthy food to young children—time to get angry, get active. *Public Health Nutrition, 12*(6), 882.

Lobstein, T., & Baur, L. (2005). Policies to prevent childhood obesity in the European Union. *European Journal of Public Health, 15*(6), 576–579.

Lobstein, T., Baur, L., & Jackson-Leach, R. (2010). The childhood obesity epidemic. In E. Waters, B. Swinburn, J. Seidell, & R. Uauy (Eds.), *Preventing childhood obesity: Evidence, policy and practice* (pp. 3–14). Oxford: Wiley-Blackwell.

Lobstein, T., & Dibb, S. (2005). Evidence of a possible link between obesogenic food advertising and child overweight. *Obesity Reviews, 6*(3), 203–208.

Lobstein, T., & Frelut, M. (2003). Prevalence of overweight among children in Europe. *Obesity Reviews, 4*(4), 195–200.

Lorenc, T., Petticrew, M., Welch, V., & Tugwell, P. (2013). What types of interventions generate inequalities? Evidence from systematic reviews. *Journal of Epidemiology and Community Health, 67*(2), 190–193.

Ludwig, D. S. (2002). The glycemic index—physiological mechanisms relating to obesity, diabetes, and cardiovascular disease. *Journal of the American Medical Association, 287*(18), 2414–2423.

Ludwig, D. S. (2007). Childhood obesity—the shape of things to come. *New England Journal of Medicine, 357*(23), 2325–2327.

Ludwig, D. S. (2012). Weight loss strategies for adolescents: A 14-year-old struggling to lose weight. *Journal of the American Medical Association, 307*(5), 498–508.

Lumeng, J. C., Appugliese, D., Cabral, H. J., Bradley, R. H., & Zuckerman, B. (2006). Neighborhood safety and overweight status in children. *Archives of Pediatrics & Adolescent Medicine, 160*(1), 25–31.

Lunner, K., Werthem, E. H., Thompson, J. K., Paxton, S. J., McDonald, F., & Halvaarson, K. S. (2000). A cross-cultural examination of weight-related teasing, body image, and eating disturbance in Swedish and Australian samples. *International Journal of Eating Disorders, 28*(4), 430–435.

Lustig, R. H., Schmidt, L. A., & Brindis, C. D. (2012). The toxic truth about sugar. *Nature, 482*(7383), 27–29.

Mackay, J., & Eriksen, M. (2002). *The tobacco atlas.* Geneva: World Health Organization. Retrieved April 8, 2013, from http://whqlibdoc.who.int/publications/2002/9241562099.pdf.

MacLean, L., Edwards, N., Garrard, M., Sims-Jones, N., Clinton, K., & Ashley, L. (2009). Obesity, stigma and public health planning. *Health Promotion International, 24*(1), 88–93.

MacLean, L., Meyer, M., Walsh, A., Clinton, K., Ashley, L., Donovan, S., & Edwards, N. (2010). Stigma and BMI screening in schools, or "Mom, I hate it when they weigh me." In J. A. O'Dea & M. Erisken (Eds.), *Childhood obesity prevention: International research, controversies, and interventions* (pp. 17–30). New York: Oxford University Press.

Magnus, A., Haby, M. M., Carter, R., & Swinburn, B. (2009). The cost-effectiveness of removing television advertising of high-fat and/or high-sugar food and beverages to Australian children. *International Journal of Obesity, 33*(10), 1094–1102.

Maher, J., Fraser, S., & Wright, J. (2010). Framing the mother: Childhood obesity, maternal responsibility and care. *Journal of Gender Studies, 19*(3), 233–247.

Major, B., & O'Brien, L. T. (2005). The social psychology of stigma. *Annual Review of Psychology, 56*(1), 393–421.

Manios, Y., & Costarelli, V. (2011). Childhood obesity in the WHO European region. In L. A. Moreno, I. Pigeot, & W. Ahrens (Eds.), *Epidemiology of obesity in children and adolescents* (pp. 43–68). New York: Springer.

Marmot, M., Friel, S., Bell, R., Houweling, T., & Taylor, S., on behalf of the Commission on Social Determinants of Health. (2008). Closing the gap in a generation: Health equity through action on the social determinants of health. *The Lancet, 372*(9650), 1661–1669.

Marmot, M., & Wilkinson, R. (Eds.). (2003). *Social determinants of health* (2nd ed.). Oxford: Oxford University Press.

Marples, R. (2002). Well-being as an aim of education. In R. Marples (Ed.), *The aims of education* (pp. 133–144). London: Routledge.

Marshall, T. (2000). Exploring a fiscal food policy: The case of diet and ischaemic heart disease. *British Medical Journal, 320*(7230), 301–305.

Martin, D. (2007, 15 June). Treat child obesity as neglect, say doctors. *Daily Mail.* Retrieved October 19, 2012, from http://www.dailymail.co.uk/news/article-461876/Treat-child-obesity-neglect-say-doctors.html.

Matheson, F. I., Moineddin, R., & Glazier, R. H. (2008). The weight of place: A multilevel analysis of gender, neighborhood material deprivation, and body mass index among Canadian adults. *Social Science & Medicine, 66*(3), 675–690.

Matthews, A. E. (2008). Children and obesity: A pan-European project examining the role of food marketing. *European Journal of Public Health, 18*(1), 7–11.

McCurdy, L. E., Winterbottom, K. E., Mehta, S. S., & Roberts, J. R. (2010). Using nature and outdoor activity to improve children's health. *Current Problems in Pediatric and Adolescent Health Care, 40*(5), 102–117.

McDermott, A. J., & Stephens, M. B. (2010). Cost of eating whole foods versus convenience foods in a low-income model. *Family Medicine, 42*(4), 280–284.

McDermott, L., O'Sullivan, T., Stead, M., & Hastings, G. (2006). International food advertising, pester power, and its effects. *International Journal of Advertising, 25*(4), 513–539.

McGeehan, P. (2011, August 19). Ban on using food stamps to buy soda rejected by USDA. *New York Times.* Retrieved May 20, 2013, from http://www.nytimes.com/2011/08/20/nyregion/ban-on-using-food-stamps-to-buy-soda-rejected-by-usda.html?_r=0.

Ménard, J.-F. (2010). A "nudge" for public health ethics: Libertarian paternalism as a framework for ethical analysis of public health interventions? *Public Health Ethics, 3*(3), 229–238.

Metcalf, B., Henley, W., & Wilkin, T. (2012). Effectiveness of intervention on physical activity of children: Systematic review and meta-analysis of controlled trials with objectively measured outcomes. *British Medical Journal, 345*, e5888.

Meyer, K. A., Wall, M. M., Larson, N. I., Laska, M. N., & Neumark-Sztainer, D. (2012). Sleep duration and BMI in a sample of young adults. *Obesity, 20*(6), 1279–1287.

Michaels, D. (2008). *Doubt is their product: How industry's assault on science threatens your health.* New York: Oxford University Press.

Mielck, A., Graham, H., & Bremberg, S. (2002). Children, an important target group for the reduction of socioeconomic inequalities in health. In J. P. Mackenbach & M. Bakker (Eds.), *Reducing inequalities in health: A European perspective* (pp. 144–168). London: Routledge.

Miller, J. C., & Coble, K. H. (2007). Cheap food policy: Fact or rhetoric? *Food Policy, 32*(1), 98–111.

Mills, C. W. (2000). *The sociological imagination.* Oxford: Oxford University Press.

Minaker, L. M., Storey, K. E., Raine, K. D., Spence, J. C., Forbes, L. E., & Plotnikoff, R. C. (2011). Associations between the perceived presence of vending machines and food and beverage logos in schools and adolescents' diet and weight status. *Public Health Nutrition, 14*(8), 1350–1356.

Ministry of Health and Social Policy of Spain. (2010). *Moving forward equity in health: Monitoring social determinants of health and the reduction of health inequalities.* Madrid: Ministry of Health and Social Policy.

Mission: Readiness—Military Leaders for Kids. (2010). *Too fat to fight: Retired military leaders want junk food out of America's schools.* New York: Mission: Readiness—Military Leaders for Kids. Retrieved February 22, 2013, from http://cdn.mission-readiness.org/MR_Too_Fat_to_Fight-1.pdf.

Mitchell, L. E. (2001). *Corporate irresponsibility: America's newest export*. New Haven, CT: Yale University Press.

Mladovsky, P., Allin, S., Masseria, C., Hernández-Quevedo, C., McDaid, D., & Mossialos, E. (2009). *Health in the European Union: Trends and analysis*. Brussels: European Observatory on Health Systems and Policies.

Mold, F., & Forbes, A. (2011). Patients' and professionals' experiences and perspectives of obesity in health-care settings: A synthesis of current research. *Health Expectations, 16*(2), 119–142.

Monteiro, C. A. (2009). Nutrition and health: The issue is not food, nor nutrients, so much as processing. *Public Health Nutrition, 12*(5), 729–731.

Monteiro, C. A. (2010). Commentary: The big issue is ultra-processing. *World Nutrition: Journal of the World Public Health Nutrition Association, 1*(6), 237–269. Retrieved April 18, 2013, from http://www.wphna.org/downloadsnovermber2010/10-11 WN Comm Food processing.pdf.

Moodie, R., Stuckler, D., Monteiro, C. A., Sheron, N., Neal, B., Thamarangsi, T., Lincoln, P., & Casswell, S., on behalf of The Lancet NCD Action Group. (2013). Profits and pandemics: Prevention of harmful effects of tobacco, alcohol, an ultra-processed food and drink industries. *The Lancet, 381*(9867), 670–679.

Moore, E. S. (2004). Children and the changing world of advertising. *Journal of Business Ethics, 52*(2), 161–167.

Mozaffarian, D., Afshin, A., Benowitz, N. L., Bittner, V., Daniels, S. R., Franch, H. A., Jacobs Jr, D. R., Kraus, W. E., Kris-Etherton, P. M., Krummel, D. A., Popkin, B. M., Whitsel, L. P., & Zakai, N. A., on behalf of the American Heart Association Council on Epidemiology and Prevention, Council on Nutrition, Physical Activity and Metabolism, Council on Clinical Cardiology, Council on Cardiovascular Disease in the Young, Council on the Kidney in Cardiovascular Disease, Council on Peripheral Vascular Disease, and the Advocacy Coordinating Committee. (2012). Population approaches to improve diet, physical activity, and smoking habits: A scientific statement from the American Heart Foundation. *Circulation, 126*(12), 1514–1563.

Muckelbauer, R., Libuda, L., Clausen, K., Toschke, A. M., Reinehr, T., & Kersting, M. (2009). Promotion and provision of drinking water in schools for overweight prevention: Randomized, controlled cluster trial. *Pediatrics, 123*(4), e661–667.

Muennig, P. (2008). The body politic: The relationship between stigma and obesity-associated disease. *BMC Public Health, 8*(1), 128.

Muennig, P., Jia, H., Lee, R., & Lubetkin, E. (2008). I think therefore I am: Perceived ideal weight as a determinant of health. *American Journal of Public Health, 98*(3), 501–506.

Muennig, P., Lubetkin, E., Jia, H., & Franks, P. (2006). Gender and the burden of disease attributable to obesity. *American Journal of Public Health, 96*(9), 1662–1668.

Muller, M., Schoonover, H., & Wallinga, D. (2007). *Considering the contribution of US food and agricultural policy to the obesity epidemic: Overview and opportunities*.

Minneapolis, MN: Institute for Agriculture and Trade Policy. Retrieved April 1, 2013, from http://www.iatp.org/files/258_2_99608.pdf.

Müller, M. J., Danielzik, S., & Pust, S. (2005). School- and family-based interventions to prevent overweight in children. *Proceedings of the Nutrition Society, 64*(2), 249–254.

Murtagh, L., & Ludwig, D. S. (2011). State intervention in life-threatening childhood obesity. *Journal of the American Medical Association, 306*(2), 206–207.

Must, A., & Anderson, S. E. (2006). Body mass index in children and adolescents: Considerations for population-based applications. *International Journal of Obesity, 30*(4), 590–594.

Mytton, O., Gray, A., Rayner, M., & Rutter, H. (2007). Could targeted food taxes improve health? *Journal of Epidemiology & Community Health, 61*(8), 689–694.

Nairn, A., & Fine, C. (2008). Who's messing with my mind? The implications of dual-process models for the ethics of advertising to children. *International Journal of Advertising, 27*(3), 447–470.

Nairn, A., Omrod, J., & Bottomley, P. (2007). *Watching, wanting and well-being: Exploring the links. A study of 9–13 year olds.* London: National Consumer Council. Retrieved April 20, 2013, from http://www.agnesnairn.co.uk/policy_reports/watching_wanting_and_wellbeing_july_2007.pdf.

Nash, C., & Basini, S. (2012). Pester power: It's all in "the game." *Young Consumers: Insight and Ideas for Responsible Marketers, 13*(3), 267–283.

National Health and Medical Research Council (Australia). (2003). *Clinical practice guidelines for the management of overweight and obesity in adults.* Canberra: National Health & Medical Research Council. Retrieved May 17, 2013, from http://www.health.gov.au/internet/main/publishing.nsf/Content/893169B10DD846FCCA256F190003BADA/$File/children.pdf.

Nestle, M. (2006). Food marketing and childhood obesity—a matter of policy. *New England Journal of Medicine, 354*(24), 2527–2529.

Neumark-Sztainer, D. (2005). *I'm, like, SO fat!: Helping your teen make healthy choices about eating and exercise in a weight-obsessed world.* New York: Guildford Press.

Neumark-Sztainer, D., Falkner, N., Story, M., Perry, C., & Hannan, P. J., & Mulert, S. (2002). Weight-teasing among adolescents: Correlations with weight status and disordered eating behaviors. *International Journal of Obesity, 26*(1), 123–131.

Neumark-Sztainer, D., Story, M., & Harris, T. (1999). Beliefs and attitudes about obesity among teachers and school health care providers working with adolescents. *Journal of Nutrition Education, 31*(1), 3–9.

Neumark-Sztainer, D., Wall, M., Larson, N. I., Eisenberg, M. E., & Loth, K. (2011). Dieting and disordered eating behaviors from adolescence to young adulthood: Findings from a 10-year longitudinal study. *Journal of the American Dietetic Association, 111*(7), 1004–1011.

Neumark-Sztainer, D., Wall, M., Story, M., & Standish, A. R. (2012). Dieting and unhealthy weight control behaviors during adolescence: Associations with 10-year changes in Body Mass Index. *Journal of Adolescent Health, 50*(1), 80–86.

Neumark-Sztainer, D., Wall, M., Story, M., & van den Berg, P. (2008). Accurate parental classification of overweight adolescents' weight status: Does it matter? *Pediatrics*, *121*(6), e1495–1502.

NHS Choices. (2010, January 9). The National Child Measurement Programme. Retrieved August 8, 2011, from http://www.nhs.uk/Livewell/childhealth1-5/Pages/ChildMeasurement.aspx.

NHS Information Centre. (2012). Obesity. Retrieved September 18, 2012, from http://www.ic.nhs.uk/statistics-and-data-collections/health-and-lifestyles/obesity.

Ni Mhurchu, C., Blakely, T., Jiang, Y., Eyles, H. C., & Rodgers, A. (2010). Effects of price discounts and tailored nutrition education on supermarket purchases: A randomized controlled trial. *The American Journal of Clinical Nutrition*, *91*(3), 736–747.

Ni Mhurchu, C., Blakely, T., Wall, J., Rodgers, A., Jiang, Y., & Wilton, J. (2007). Strategies to promote healthier food purchases: A pilot supermarket intervention study. *Public Health Nutrition*, *10*(6), 608–615.

Nicholls, S. G. (2013). Standards and classification: A perspective on the "obesity epidemic." *Social Science & Medicine*, *87*, 9–15.

Nicholls, S. G., Gwozdz, W., Reisch, L., & Voigt, K. (2011a). Fiscal food policy: Equity and practice. *Perspectives in Public Health*, *131*(4), 157–158.

Nicholls, S. G., Voigt, K., Siani, A., De Henauw, S., Marild, S., Molnár, D., Moreno, L. A., Tornaritis, M., Veidebaum, T., Pigeot, I., & Ahrens, W. (2011b). Price strategies and health inequalities: Support for taxation of unhealthy foods among low-income groups in European countries. Paper presented at Promoting Health Equity: Action on the Social Determinants of Health, Toronto, Canada.

Niederdeppe, J., Fiore, M. C., Baker, T. B., & Smith, S. S. (2008). Smoking-cessation media campaigns and their effectiveness among socioeconomically advantaged and disadvantaged populations. *American Journal of Public Health*, *98*(5), 916–924.

Nnoaham, K. E., Sacks, G., Rayner, M., Mytton, O., & Gray, A. (2009). Modelling income group differences in the health and economic impacts of targeted food taxes and subsidies. *International Journal of Epidemiology*, *38*(5), 1324–1333.

Noggle, R. (2002). Special agents: Children's autonomy and parental authority. In D. Archard & C. Macleod (Eds.). *The moral and political status of children* (pp. 97–117). Oxford: Oxford University Press.

Norheim, O. F. (2009). Implementing the Marmot Commission's recommendations: Social justice requires a solution to the equity-efficiency trade-off. *Public Health Ethics*, *2*(1), 53–58.

Nutley, S. (2003). Bridging the policy/research divide: Reflections and lessons from the UK. Retrieved May 8, 2013, from http://www.st-andrews.ac.uk/~ruruweb/pdf/Bridging Research Policy Divide.pdf.

Nys, T. R. V. (2008). Paternalism in public health care. *Public Health Ethics*, *1*(1), 64–72.

O'Brien, K. S., Hunter, J. A., & Banks, M. (2006). Implicit anti-fat bias in physical educators: Physical attributes, ideology and socialization. *International Journal of Obesity*, *31*(2), 308–314.

O'Connor, D. (2013, January 25). Dan Callahan thinsplains obesity. Retrieved March 1, 2013, from http://bioethicsbulletin.org/archive/dan-callahan-thinsplains-obesity/.

O'Dea, J. A. (2005). Prevention of childhood obesity: "First, do no harm." *Health Education Research, 20*(2), 259–265.

O'Dea, J. A. (2010). Developing positive approaches to nutrition education and the prevention of child and adolescent obesity: First, do no harm. In J. O'Dea & M. Eriksen (Eds.), *Childhood obesity prevention: International research, controversies, and interventions* (pp. 31–41). New York: Oxford University Press.

O'Dea, J. A., & Eriksen, M. (Eds.). (2010). *Childhood obesity prevention: International research, controversies, and interventions.* New York: Oxford University Press.

O'Dea, J. A., & Wilson, R. (2006). Socio-cognitive and nutritional factors associated with body mass index in children and adolescents: Possibilities for childhood obesity prevention. *Health Education Research, 21*(6), 796–805.

O'Neill, O. (1998). Instituting principles: Between duty and action. *The Southern Journal of Philosophy, 36*(Supplement), 79–96; reprinted in M. Timmons (Ed.), *Kant's metaphysics of morals: Interpretive essays* (pp. 331–347). Oxford: Oxford University Press.

O'Neill, O. (2002). *Autonomy and trust in bioethics.* Cambridge: Cambridge University Press.

O'Neill, O. (2004). Modern moral philosophy and the problem of relevant descriptions. *Royal Institute of Philosophy Supplement, 54*(1), 301–316.

O'Neill, O. (2007). Normativity and practical judgement. *Journal of Moral Philosophy, 4*(3), 393–405.

OECD. (2012). *Obesity update 2012.* Paris: Organisation for Economic Co-operation and Development. Retrieved September 14, 2012, from http://www.oecd.org/els/healthpoliciesanddata/49716427.pdf.

Ofcom. (2007). Television advertising of food and drink products to children: Final statement. London: Great Britain Office of Communications. Retrieved March 7, 2013, from http://stakeholders.ofcom.org.uk/binaries/consultations/foodads_new/statement/statement.pdf.

Ofcom. (2010). *HFSS advertising restrictions: Final review.* London: Great Britain Office of Communications. Retrieved April 19, 2011, from http://stakeholders.ofcom.org.uk/binaries/research/tv-research/hfss-review-final.pdf.

Ogden, C. L., Carroll, M. D., & Flegal, K. M. (2010). A review of prevalence and trends in childhood obesity in the United States. In J. A. O'Dea & M. Erisken (Eds.), *Childhood obesity prevention: International research, controversies, and interventions* (pp. 84–94). New York: Oxford University Press.

Ogden, C. L., Carroll, M. D., Kit, B. K., & Flegal, K. M. (2012). Prevalence of obesity and trends in body mass index among us children and adolescents, 1999–2010. *Journal of the American Medical Association, 307*(5), 483–490.

Okonkwo, O., & While, A. (2010). University students' views of obesity and weight management strategies. *Health Education Journal, 69*(2), 192–199.

Okrent, A. M., & Alston, J. M. (2012). The effects of farm commodity and retail food policies on obesity and economic welfare in the United States. *American Journal of Agricultural Economics, 94*(3), 611–646.

Oliver, J. E. (2006). *Fat politics: The real story behind America's obesity epidemic.* Oxford: Oxford University Press.

Oliver, J. E., & Lee, T. (2005). Public opinion and the politics of obesity in America. *Journal of Health Politics, Policy and Law, 30*(5), 923–954.

Olshansky, S. J., Passaro, D. J., Hershow, R. C., Layden, J., Carnes, B. A., Brody, J., Hayflick, L., Butler, R. N., Allison, D. B., & Ludwig, D. S. (2005). A potential decline in life expectancy in the United States in the 21st century. *New England Journal of Medicine, 352*(11), 1138–1145.

Ortega, F. B., Lee, D. C., Katzmarzyk, P. T., Ruiz, J. R., Sui, X., Church, T. S., & Blair, S. N. (2013). The intriguing metabolically healthy but obese phenotype: Cardiovascular prognosis and role of fitness. *European Heart Journal, 34*(5), 389–397.

Page, R. M., & Brewster, A. (2007). Emotional and rational product appeals in televised food advertisements for children: Analysis of commercials shown on US broadcast networks. *Journal of Child Health Care, 11*(4), 323–340.

Pantenburg, B., Sikorski, C., Luppa, M., Schomerus, G., König, H.-H., Werner, P., & Riedel-Heller, S. G. (2012). Medical students' attitudes towards overweight and obesity. *PLoS ONE, 7*(11), e48113.

Papas, M. A., Alberg, A. J., Ewing, R., Helzlsouer, K. J., Gary, T. L., & Klassen, A. C. (2007). The built environment and obesity. *Epidemiologic Reviews, 29*(1), 129–143.

Park, M. H., Falconer, C., Viner, R. M., & Kinra, S. (2012). The impact of childhood obesity on morbidity and mortality in adulthood: A systematic review. *Obesity Reviews, 13*(11), 985–1000.

Perry, J. (2007, May 25). Motion. City of Los Angeles. Retrieved April 4, 2013, from http://clkrep.lacity.org/onlinedocs/2007/07–1658_mot_5–25–07.pdf.

Peterson, K. E., & Fox, M. K. (2007). Addressing the epidemic of childhood obesity through school-based interventions: What has been done and where do we go from here? *The Journal of Law, Medicine & Ethics, 35*(1), 113–130.

Phipps, S., Burton, P., Osberg, L., & Lethbridge, L. (2006). Poverty and the extent of child obesity in Canada, Norway and the United States. *Obesity Reviews, 7*(1), 5–12.

Piran, N., Levine, M., & Irving, L. (2000). GO GIRLS! Media literacy, activism, and advocacy project. *Healthy Weight Journal, 14*(6), 89–90.

Pogge, T. W. (2002). Responsibilities for poverty related ill health. *Ethics and International Affairs, 16*(2), 71–79.

Pollan, M. (2008). *In defense of food: An eater's manifesto.* New York: Penguin.

Popkin, B. M. (2011). Agricultural policies, food and public health. *EMBO Reports, 12*(1), 11–18.

Potestio, M. L., McLaren, L., Vollman, A. R., & Dole-Baker, P. K. (2008). Childhood obesity: Perceptions held by the public in Calgary, Canada. *Canadian Journal of Public Health-Revue Canadienne de Santé Publique, 99*(2), 86–90.

Powell, L. M., & Chaloupka, F. J. (2009). Food prices and obesity: Evidence and policy implications for taxes and subsidies. *The Milbank Quarterly, 87*(1), 229–257.

Powell, L. M., Chriqui, J., & Chaloupka, F. J. (2009). Associations between state-level soda taxes and adolescent Body Mass Index. *Journal of Adolescent Health, 45*(3 Supplement), s57–s63.

Powell, L. M., Szczypka, G., Chaloupka, F. J., & Braunschweig, C. L. (2007). Nutritional content of television food advertisements seen by children and adolescents in the United States. *Pediatrics, 120*(3), 576–583.

Power, C., Lake, J. K., & Cole, T. J. (1997). Measurement and long-term health risks of child and adolescent fatness. *International Journal of Obesity, 21*(7), 507–526.

Power, C., Manor, O., & Matthews, S. (2003). Child to adult socioeconomic conditions and obesity in a national cohort. *International Journal of Obesity, 27*(9), 1081–1086.

Preston, C. (2004). Children's advertising: The ethics of economic socialization. *International Journal of Consumer Studies, 28*(4), 364–370.

Puhl, R. M., & Brownell, K. D. (2001). Bias, discrimination and obesity. *Obesity Research, 9*(12), 788–805.

Puhl, R. M., & Heuer, C. A. (2009). The stigma of obesity: A review and update. *Obesity, 17*(5), 941–964.

Puhl, R. M., & Heuer, C. (2010). Obesity stigma: Important considerations for public health. *American Journal of Public Health, 100*(6), 1019–1028.

Puhl, R. M., & Latner, J. D. (2007). Stigma, obesity, and the health of the nation's children. *Psychological Bulletin, 133*(4), 557–580.

Putnam, J., Allshouse, J., & Scott Kantor, L. (2003). US per capita food supply trends: More calories, refined carbohydrates, and fats. *Food Review, 25*(3), 2–15.

Quick, V., Wall, M., Larson, N., Haines, J., & Neumark-Sztainer, D. (2013). Personal, behavioral and socio-environmental predictors of overweight incidence in young adults: 10-year longitudinal findings. *International Journal of Behavioral Nutrition and Physical Activity, 10*(1), 37.

Rampersaud, G., Pereira, M., Girard, B., Adams, J., & Metzl, J. (2005). Breakfast habits, nutritional status, body weight, and academic performance in children and adolescents. *Journal of the American Dietetic Association, 105*(5), 743–760.

Randolph, W., & Viswanath, K. (2004). Lessons learned from public health mass media campaigns: Marketing health in a crowded media world. *Annual Review of Public Health, 25*, 419–437.

Raudenbush, S. W., & Bryk, A. S. (2002). *Hierarchical linear models* (2nd ed.). Thousand Oaks, CA: Sage.

Rawls, J. (1973). *A theory of justice*. New York: Oxford University Press.

Reilly, J. J. (2006). Diagnostic accuracy of the BMI for age in pediatrics. *International Journal of Obesity, 30*(4), 595–597.

Reilly, J. J., Methven, E., McDowell, Z., Hacking, B., Alexander, D., Stewart, L., & Kelnar, C. (2003). Health consequences of obesity. *Archives of Disease in Childhood, 88*(9), 748–752.

Richardson, H. S. (2000). The stupidity of the cost-benefit standard. *Journal of Legal Studies*, *29*(S2), 971–1003.

Richardson, H. S. (2004). *Democratic autonomy: Public reasoning about the ends of policy*. New York: Oxford University Press.

Richardson, S. A., Goodman, N., Hastorf, A. H., & Dornbusch, S. M. (1961). Cultural uniformity in reaction to physical disabilities. *American Sociological Review*, *26*(2), 241–247.

Ripstein, A. (1999). *Equality, responsibility and the law*. Cambridge: Cambridge University Press.

Ripstein, A. (2009). *Force and freedom: Kant's legal and political philosophy*. Cambridge: Harvard University Press.

Rittel, H. W. J., & Webber, M. M. (1973). Dilemmas in a general theory of planning. *Policy Sciences*, *4*(2), 155–169.

Roberts, D. F. (1983). Children and commercials: Issues, evidence, interventions. *Prevention in Human Services*, *2*(1–2), 19–35.

Roberts, P. (2008). *The end of food*. Boston: Houghton Mifflin Harcourt.

Robertson, A., Lobstein, T., & Knai, C. (2007). *Obesity and socio-economic groups in Europe: Evidence review and implications for action*. Brussels: European Commission. Retrieved February 22, 2013, from http://ec.europa.eu/health/ph_determinants/life_style/nutrition/documents/ev20081028_rep_en.pdf.

Robinson, T. N. (2010). Save the world, prevent obesity: Piggybacking on existing social and ideological movements. *Obesity*, *18*(Supplement 1), S17–S22.

Rodríguez, G., Pietrobelli, A., Wang, Y., & Moreno, L. A. (2011). Methodological aspects for childhood and adolescence obesity epidemiology. In L. A. Moreno, I. Pigeot, & W. Ahrens (Eds.), *Epidemiology of obesity in children and adolescents* (pp. 21–40). New York: Springer.

Rokholm, B., Baker, J. L., & Sørensen, T. I. A. (2010). The levelling off of the obesity epidemic since the year 1999—a review of evidence and perspectives. *Obesity Reviews*, *11*(12), 835–846.

Rose, G. (1992). *The strategy of preventive medicine*. Oxford: Oxford University Press.

Ross, B. (2005). Fat or fiction: Weighing the "obesity epidemic." In M. Gard & J. Wright (Eds.), *The obesity epidemic: Science, morality and ideology* (pp. 86–106). London: Routledge.

Rozin, P. (1997). Moralization. In A. Brandt & P. Rozin (Eds.), *Morality and health* (pp. 379–401). New York: Routledge.

Rudd Center for Food Policy & Obesity. (2009). *Soft drink taxes: Opportunities for public policy*. New Haven, CT: Rudd Center for Food Policy & Obesity. Retrieved April 8, 2013, from http://www.docstoc.com/docs/28143702/Yale-Rudd-Center-Soft-Drink-Tax-Report-Feb-2009.

Rutter, H. (2012). The single most important intervention to tackle obesity. *International Journal of Public Health*, *57*(4), 657–658.

Sacks, G., Swinburn, B., & Lawrence, M. (2009). Obesity Policy Action framework and analysis grids for a comprehensive policy approach to reducing obesity. *Obesity Reviews, 10*(1), 78–86.

Sacks, G., Veerman, J. L., Moodie, M., & Swinburn, B. (2011). "Traffic-light" nutrition labelling and "junk-food" tax: A modelled comparison of cost-effectiveness for obesity prevention. *International Journal of Obesity, 35*(7), 1001–1009.

Saelens, B. E., Sallis, J. F., Frank, L. D., Couch, S. C., Zhou, C., Colburn, T., Cain, K. L., Chapman, J., & Glanz, K. (2012). Obesogenic neighborhood environments, child and parent obesity: The Neighborhood Impact on Kids study. *American Journal of Preventive Medicine, 42*(5), e57–e64.

Saguy, A. C., & Almeling, R. (2008). Fat in the fire? Science, the news media, and the "obesity epidemic." *Sociological Forum, 23*(1), 53–83.

Sahota, P., Rudolf, M. C. J., Dixey, R., Hill, A. J., Barth, J. H., & Cade, J. E. (2001). Evaluation of implementation and effect of primary school based intervention to reduce risk factors for obesity. *British Medical Journal, 323*(7320), 1027–1029.

Saletan, W. (2008, July 31). Food apartheid: Banning fast food in poor neighborhoods. *Slate*. Retrieved May 25, 2013, from http://www.slate.com/articles/health_and_science/human_nature/2008/07/food_apartheid.html.

Sallis, J. F., & Glanz, K. (2006). The role of built environments in physical activity, eating, and obesity in childhood. *Future of Children, 16*(1), 89–108.

Saxena, S., Ambler, G., Cole, T., & Majeed, A. (2004). Ethnic group differences in overweight and obese children and young people in England: Cross sectional survey. *Archives of Disease in Childhood, 89*(1), 30–36.

Scarre, G. (1980). Children and paternalism. *Philosophy, 55*(211), 117–124.

Schinkel, A., de Ruyter, D., & Steutel, J. (2010). Threats to autonomy in consumer societies and their implications for education. *Theory and Research in Education, 8*(3), 269–287.

Schroeter, C., Lusk, J., & Tyner, W. (2008). Determining the impact of food price and income changes on body weight. *Journal of Health Economics, 27*(1), 45–68.

Schwartz, M. B., & Brownell, K. D. (2007). Actions necessary to prevent childhood obesity: Creating the climate for change. *Journal of Law, Medicine, and Ethics, 35*(1), 78–89.

Schwartz, M. B., & Puhl, R. M. (2003). Childhood obesity: A societal problem to solve. *Obesity Reviews, 4*(1), 57–71.

Segall, S. (2009). *Health, luck, and justice*. Princeton, NJ: Princeton University Press.

Shenkin, J. D., & Jacobson, M. F. (2010). Using the food stamp program and other methods to promote healthy diets for low-income consumers. *American Journal of Public Health, 100*(9), 1562–1564.

Sherwell, P. (2008, July 26). Los Angeles bans new fast food outlets and California outlaws trans-fats. *Daily Telegraph*. Retrieved May 25, 2013, from http://www.telegraph.co.uk/news/worldnews/northamerica/usa/2461615/Los-Angeles-bans-new-fast-food-outlets-and-California-outlaws-trans-fats.html.

Sherwin, J. C., Reacher, M. H., Keogh, R. H., Khawaja, A. P., Mackey, D. A., & Foster, P. J. (2012). The association between time spent outdoors and myopia in children and adolescents: A systematic review and meta-analysis. *Ophthalmology, 119*(10), 2141–2151.

Siahpush, M., Wakefield, M., A. Spittal, M. J., Durkin, S. J., & Scollo, M. M. (2009). Taxation reduces social disparities in adult smoking prevalence. *American Journal of Preventive Medicine, 36*(4), 285–291.

Sichert-Hellert, W., Berghin, L., De Henauw, S., Grammatikaki, E., Hallström, L., Manios, Y., Mesana, M. I., Molnár, D., Dietrich, S., Piccinelli, R., Plada, M., Sjöström, M., Moreno, L. A., & Kersting, M., on behalf of the HELENA study group. (2011). Nutritional knowledge in European adolescents: Results from the HELENA (Healthy Lifestyle in Europe by Nutrition in Adolescence) study. *Public Health Nutrition, 14*(12), 2083–2091.

Singh, A. S., Mulder, C., Twisk, J. W., van Mechelen, W., & Chinapaw, M. J. (2008). Tracking of childhood overweight into adulthood: A systematic review of the literature. *Obesity Reviews, 9*(5), 474–488.

Singh, G. K., Kogan, M. D., Van Dyck, P. C., & Siahpush, M. (2008). Racial/ethnic, socioeconomic, and behavioral determinants of childhood and adolescent obesity in the United States: Analyzing independent and joint associations. *Annals of Epidemiology, 18*(9), 682–695.

Skatrud-Mickelson, M., Adachi-Mejia, A. M., MacKenzie, T. A., & Sutherland, L. A. (2012). Giving the wrong impression: Food and beverage brand impressions delivered to youth through popular movies. *Journal of Public Health, 34*(2), 245–252.

Slater, A., Bowen, J., Corsini, N., Gardner, C., Golley, R., & Noakes, M. (2009). Understanding parent concerns about children's diet, activity and weight status: An important step towards effective obesity prevention interventions. *Public Health Nutrition, 13*(8), 1221–1228.

Smalley, K. J., Knerr, A. N., Kendrick, Z. V., Colliver, J. A., & Owen, O. E. (1990). Reassessment of body mass indices. *American Journal of Clinical Nutrition, 52(3)*, 405–408.

Song, Y., Park, M. J., Paik, H. Y., & Joung, H. (2009). Secular trends in dietary patterns and obesity-related risk factors in Korean adolescents aged 10–19 years. *International Journal of Obesity, 34*(1), 48–56.

Speers, S. E., Harris, J. L., & Schwartz, M. B. (2011). Child and adolescent exposure to food and beverage brand appearances during prime-time television programming. *American Journal of Preventive Medicine, 41*(3), 291–296.

Spencer, S. J., Steele, C. M., & Quinn, D. M. (1999). Stereotype threat and women's math performance. *Journal of Experimental Social Psychology, 35*(1), 4–28.

Stamatakis, E., Primatesta, P., Chinn, S., Rona, R., & Falascheti, E. (2005). Overweight and obesity trends from 1974 to 2003 in English children: What is the role of socio-economic factors? *Archives of Disease in Childhood, 90*(10), 999–1004.

Stead, M., McDermott, L., & Hastings, G. (2007). Towards evidence-based marketing: The case of childhood obesity. *Marketing Theory, 7*(4), 379–406.

Stead, M., McDermott, L., MacKintosh, A. M., & Adamson, A. (2011). Why healthy eating is bad for young people's health: Identity, belonging and food. *Social Science & Medicine, 72*(7), 1131–1139.

Steele, C., & Aronson, J. (1995). Stereotype threat and the intellectual test performance of African Americans. *Journal of Personality and Social Psychology, 69*(5), 797–811.

Steinberger, J., Daniels, S. R., Eckel, R. H., Hayman, L., Lustig, R. H., McCrindle, B., & Mietus-Snyder, M. L. (2009). Progress and challenges in metabolic syndrome in children and adolescents: A scientific statement from the American Heart Association. *Circulation, 119*(4), 628–647.

Stodell, H. (2010, August 7). FSA-friendly Coco Pops launched by Kellogg's. *The Grocer.* Retrieved May 5, 2013, from http://www.thegrocer.co.uk/fmcg/fsa-friendly-c oco-pops-launches-by-kelloggs/211626.article.

Stones, M. (2012, October 26). Asda boss in PR gaffe: When radio interviews turn nasty. Retrieved January 10, 2013, from http://www.foodmanufacture.co.uk/ Food-Safety/Asda-boss-in-PR-gaffe-when-radio-interviews-turn-nasty.

Story, M., Kaphingst, K. M., & French, S. (2006). The role of schools in obesity prevention. *Future of Children, 16*(1), 109–142.

Story, M., Nanney, M. S., & Schwartz, M. B. (2009). Schools and obesity prevention: Creating school environments and policies to promote healthy eating and physical activity. *Milbank Quarterly, 87*(1), 71–100.

Strauss, R. S. (2000). Childhood obesity and self-esteem. *Pediatrics, 105*(1), e15.

Strauss, R. S., & Mir, H. M. (2001). Smoking and weight loss attempts in overweight and normal-weight adolescents. *International Journal of Obesity, 25*(9), 1381–1385.

Strauss, R. S., & Pollack, H. A. (2003). Social marginalization of overweight children. *Archives of Pediatrics & Adolescent Medicine, 157*(8), 746–752.

Strnad, J. (2004). Conceptualizing the fat tax: The role of food taxes in developed economies. *Southern California Law Review, 78*, 1221–1326.

Strom, S. (2012, November 12). "Fat tax" in Denmark is repealed after criticism. *The New York Times* (online). Retrieved February 25, 2013, from http://www.nytimes. com/2012/11/13/business/global/fat-tax-in-denmark-is-repealed-after-criticism. html?_r=0.

Stuber, J., Meyer, I., & Link, B. (2008). Stigma, prejudice, discrimination and health. *Social Science & Medicine, 67*(3), 351–357.

Stuckler, D., & Siegel, K. (2011). *Sick societies: Responding to the global challenge of chronic disease.* Oxford: Oxford University Press.

Stunkard, A. J., & Sørensen, T. I. A. (1993). Obesity and socioeconomic status—a complex relation. *New England Journal of Medicine, 329*(14), 1036–1037.

Sturm, R., & Cohen, D. A. (2009). Zoning for health? The year-old ban on new fast-food restaurants in South LA. *Health Affairs, 28*(6), w1088–w1097.

Sturm, R., & Datar, A. (2010). Regional price differences and food consumption frequency among elementary school children. *Public Health, 125*(3), 136–141.

Suggs, L. S., & McIntyre, C. (2011). European Union public opinion on policy measures to address childhood overweight and obesity. *Journal of Public Health Policy, 32*(1), 91–106.

Summerbell, C. D., Waters, E., Edmunds, L., Kelly, S. A. M., Brown, T., & Campbell, K. J. (2005). Interventions for preventing obesity in children. *Cochrane Database of Systematic Reviews* (Issue 3, Art. No.: CD001871).

Sundquist, J., & Winkleby, M. (2000). Country of birth, acculturation status and abdominal obesity in a national sample of Mexican-American women and men. *International Journal of Epidemiology, 29*(3), 470–477.

Sunstein, C., & Thaler, R. (2008). *Nudge: Improving decisions about health, wealth, and happiness.* New Haven, CT: Yale University Press.

Sutherland, L. A., MacKenzie, T., Purvis, L. A., & Dalton, M. (2010). Prevalence of food and beverage brands in movies: 1996–2005. *Pediatrics, 125*(3), 468–474.

Swinburn, B. (2008). Obesity prevention: The role of policies, laws and regulations. *Australia and New Zealand Health Policy, 5*, 12.

Swinburn, B. (2009). Closing the disparity gaps in obesity. *International Journal of Epidemiology, 38*(2), 509–511.

Swinburn, B., & Egger, G. (2002). Preventive strategies against weight gain and obesity. *Obesity Reviews, 3*(4), 289–301.

Swinburn, B., Egger, G., & Raza, F. (1999). Dissecting obesogenic environments: The development and application of a framework for identifying and prioritizing environmental interventions for obesity. *Preventive Medicine, 29*(6), 563–570.

Szwarc, S. (2004). Putting facts over fears: Examining childhood anti-obesity initiatives. *International Quarterly of Community Health Education, 23*(2), 97–116.

Taber, D. R., Chriqui, J. F., Powell, L. M., & Chaloupka, F. J. (2012). Banning all sugar-sweetened beverages in middle schools: Reduction of in-school access and purchasing but not overall consumption. *Archives of Pediatrics and Adolescent Medicine, 166*(3), 256–262.

Tajfel, H. (1981). *Human groups and social categories.* Cambridge: Cambridge University Press.

Te Velde, S. J., Brug, J., Wind, M., Hildonen, C., Bjelland, M., Pérez-Rodrigo, C., & Klepp, K.–I. (2008). Effects of a comprehensive fruit- and vegetable-promoting school-based intervention in three European countries: The Pro Children Study. *British Journal of Nutrition, 99*(4), 893–903.

Temple, N. J., Steyn, N. P., Fourie, J., & De Villiers, A. (2010). Price and availability of healthy food: A study in rural South Africa. *Nutrition, 27*(1), 55–58.

Thatcher, M. (1987). Interview for *Women's Own.* Retrieved October 10, 2012, from http://www.margaretthatcher.org/document/106689.

Trasande, L., Attina, T. M., & Blustein, J. (2012). Association between urinary bisphenol A concentration and obesity prevalence in children and adolescents. *The Journal of the American Medical Association, 308*(11), 1113–1121.

Travers, J., & Benoit-Guyod, S. (2012, June 22). Fat tax: The idea makes its way around Europe. *Myeurop.Info*. Retrieved February 25, 2013, from http://en.myeurop. info/2012/06/22/fat-tax-idea-makes-its-way-around-europe-5608.

Union of Concerned Scientists. (2012). *Heads they win tails we lose: How corporations corrupt science at the public's expense*. Cambridge, MA: Union of Concerned Scientists Publications. Retrieved March 7, 2013, from http://www.ucsusa.org/scientific_integrity/abuses_of_science/how-corporations-corrupt-science.html.

United States Department of Agriculture Economic Research Service. (2012). *Sugar & sweeteners policy*. Retrieved October 28, 2012, from http://www.ers.usda.gov/topics/crops/sugar-sweeteners/policy.aspx.

Unkrich, L. (Director). (2010). *Toy story 3* [film]. USA: Pixar.

Uretsky, S., Messerli, F. H., Bangalore, S., Champion, A., Cooper-Dehoff, R. M., Zhou, Q., & Pepine, C. J. (2007). Obesity paradox in patients with hypertension and coronary artery disease. *The American Journal of Medicine, 120*(10), 863–870.

van Baal, P. H. M., Polder, J. J., de Wit, G. A., Hoogenveen, R. T., Feenstra, T. L., Boshuizen, H. C., Engelfriet, P. M., & Brouwer, W. B. F. (2008). Lifetime medical costs of obesity: Prevention no cure for increasing health expenditure. *PLoS Medicine, 5*(2), e29: 0242–0249.

Van Dyck, D., De Meester, F., Cardon, G., Deforche, B., & De Bourdeaudhuij, I. (2013). Physical environmental attributes and active transportation in Belgium: What about adults and adolescents living in the same neighborhoods? *American Journal of Health Promotion, 27*(5), 330–338.

Varness, T., Allen, D. B., Carrel, A. L., & Fost, N. (2009). Childhood obesity and medical neglect. *Pediatrics, 123*(1), 399–406.

Vartanian, L. R., Schwartz, M. B., & Brownell, K. D. (2007). Effects of soft drink consumption on nutrition and health: A systematic review and meta-analysis. *American Journal of Public Health, 97*(4), 667–675.

Veerman, J. L., Barendregt, J. J., & Mackenbach, J. (2006). The European Common Agricultural Policy on fruits and vegetables: Exploring potential health gain from reform. *European Journal of Public Health, 16*(1), 31–35.

Veugelers, P. J., & Fitzgerald, A. L. (2005). Effectiveness of school programs in preventing childhood obesity: A multilevel comparison. *American Journal of Public Health, 95*(3), 432–435.

Vick, K. (2008, July 13). LA official wants a change of menu. *The Washington Post*. Retrieved April 4, 2013, from http://www.washingtonpost.com/wp-dyn/content/article/2008/07/12/AR2008071201557.html.

Villanueva, T. (2011). European nations launch tax attack on unhealthy foods. *Canadian Medical Association Journal, 183*(17), E1229–E1230.

Viner, R. M., Roche, E., Maguire, S. A., & Nicholls, D. E. (2010). Childhood protection and obesity: Framework for practice. *British Medical Journal, 341*, c3074.

Voss, L. D., Metcalf, B., Jeffery, A. N., & Wilkin, T. J. (2006). IOTF thresholds for overweight and obesity and their relation to metabolic risk in children. *International Journal of Obesity, 30*(4), 606–609.

Wahba, P. (2010, March 8). New York governor defends soda tax. Retrieved October 11, 2012, from http://www.reuters.com/article/2010/03/08/us-newyork-tax-s-idUSTRE6275ZU20100308.

Wallinga, D. (2010). Agricultural policy and childhood obesity: A food systems and public health commentary. *Health Affairs*, 29(3), 405–410.

Walls, H. L., Backholer, K., Proietto, J., & McNeil, J. J. (2012). Obesity and trends in life expectancy. *Journal of Obesity*, *Article ID 107989*.

Wang, Y., & Lobstein, T. (2006). Worldwide trends in childhood overweight and obesity. *International Journal of Pediatric Obesity*, 1(1), 11–25.

Wang, Y. C., McPherson, K., & Marsh, T. (2011). Health and economic burden of the projected obesity trends in the USA and the UK. *The Lancet*, 378(9793), 815–825.

Warner, K. E. (2000). The economics of tobacco: Myths and realities. *Tobacco Control*, 9(1), 78–89.

Warner, M. (2010, March 25). The soda tax wars are back: Brace yourself. *CBSNews.com*. Retrieved February 25, 2013, from http://www.cbsnews.com/8301-505123_162-44040474/the-soda-tax-wars-are-back-brace-yourself.

Waterlander, W. E., de Mul, A., Schuit, A. J., Seidell, J. C., & Steenhuis, I. H. M. (2010). Perceptions on the use of pricing strategies to stimulate healthy eating among residents of deprived neighbourhoods: A focus group study. *International Journal of Behavioral Nutrition and Physical Activity*, 7, 44.

Weiss, R., Dziuria, J., Burgert, T. S., Tamborlane, W. V., Taksali, S. E., Yeckel, C. W., Allen, K., Lopes, M., Savoye, M., Morrison, J., Sherwin, R. S., & Caprio, S. (2004). Obesity and the metabolic syndrome in children and adolescents. *New England Journal of Medicine*, 350(23), 2362–2374.

West, D. S., Raczynski, J. M., Phillips, M. M., Bursac, Z., Heath Gauss, C., & Montgomery, B. E. E. (2008). Parental recognition of overweight in school-age children. *Obesity*, 16(3), 630–636.

Westwood, M., Fayter, D., Hartley, S., Rithalia, A., Butler, G., Glasziou, P., Bland, M., Nixon, J., Stirk, L., & Rudolf, M. (2007). Childhood obesity: Should primary school children be routinely screened? A systematic review and discussion of the evidence. *Archives of Disease in Childhood*, 92(5), 416–422.

Whatley Blum, J. E., Davee, A. M., Beaudoin, C. M., Jenkins, P. L., Kaley, L. A., & Wigand, D. A. (2008). Reduced availability of sugar-sweetened beverages and diet soda has a limited impact on beverage consumption patterns in Maine high school youth. *Journal of Nutrition Education and Behaviour*, 40(6), 341–347.

Whitaker, R. C., Wright, J. A., Pepe, M. S., Seidel, K. S., & Dietz, W. H. (1997). Predicting obesity in young adulthood from childhood and parental obesity. *The New England Journal of Medicine*, 337(13), 869–873.

Whitehead, M. (1990). *The concepts and principles of equity in health*. Copenhagen: World Health Organization.

Whitehead, M. (1991). The concepts and principles of equity and health. *Health Promotion International*, 6(3), 217–228.

Wickins-Drazilova, D., & Williams, G. (2011). Ethics and public policy. In L. Moreno, I. Pigeot, & W. Ahrens (Eds.), *Epidemiology of obesity in children and adolescents: Prevalence and etiology* (pp. 7–20). New York: Springer.

Widhalm, K., Schönegger, K., Huemer, C., & Auterith, A. (2001). Does the BMI reflect body fat in obese children and adolescents? A study using the TOBEC method. *International Journal of Obesity, 25*(2), 279–285.

Wilding, J. (2012). Are the causes of obesity primarily environmental? Yes. *British Medical Journal, 345*, e5843.

Will, B., Zeeb, H., & Baune, B. (2005). Overweight and obesity at school entry among migrant and German children: A cross-sectional study. *BMC Public Health, 5*, 45.

Williams, G. (2006). "Infrastructures of responsibility": The moral tasks of institutions. *Journal of Applied Philosophy, 23*(2), 207–221.

Williams, G. (2008). Responsibility as a virtue. *Ethical Theory and Moral Practice, 11*(4), 455–470.

Williams, G. (2012a). Between ethics and right: Kantian politics and democratic purposes. *European Journal of Philosophy, 20*(3), 479–486.

Williams, G. (2012b). Responsibility. In R. Chadwick (Ed.), *Encyclopedia of applied ethics* (vol. 3, pp. 821–828). San Diego: Academic Press.

Williams, G., & Chadwick, R. (2012). Responsibilities for healthcare: Kantian reflections. *Cambridge Quarterly of Healthcare Ethics, 21*(2), 155–165.

Williams, P., Green, R., Millar, N., Frank, L., & Hartleib, R. (2007). *Working together to build food security in Nova Scotia: Participatory food costing 2004/05*. Halifax, Nova Scotia: Atlantic Health Promotion Research Centre.

Wilson, J. (2011). Why it's time to stop worrying about paternalism in health policy. *Public Health Ethics, 4*(3), 269–279.

Wilson, N., & Thomson, G. (2005). Tobacco tax as a health protecting policy: A brief review of the New Zealand evidence. *New Zealand Medical Journal, 118*(1213), 1–10.

Womack, C. A. (2012). Public health and obesity: When a pound of prevention really is worth an ounce of cure. *Public Health Ethics, 5*(3), 222–228.

Wong, F., Huhman, M., Heitzler, C., Asbury, L., Bretthauer-Mueller, R., McCarthy, S., & Londe, P. (2004). VERB™—a social marketing campaign to increase physical activity among youth. *Preventing Chronic Disease, 1*(3), A10.

Wong, Y., Chang, Y.-J., Tsai, M.-R., Liu, T.-W., & Lin, W. (2011). The body image, weight satisfaction, and eating disorder tendency of school children: The 2-year follow up study. *Journal of the American College of Nutrition, 30*(2), 126–133.

Woo, J. G., Dolan, L. M., Morrow, A. L., Geraghty, S. R., & Goodman, E. (2008). Breastfeeding helps explain racial and socioeconomic status disparities in adolescent adiposity. *Pediatrics, 121*(3), e458-e465.

Woodman, J., Thomas, J., & Dickson, K. (2012). How explicable are differences between reviews that appear to address a similar research question? A review of reviews of physical activity interventions. *Systematic Reviews, 1*, article number 37.

World Health Organization. (2007). *Ethical considerations in developing a public health response to pandemic influenza*. Geneva: World Health Organization.

World Health Organization. (2010). *Urban HEART—Urban Health Equity Assessment and Response Tool.* Kobe: World Health Organization.

Wright, C. M., Parker, L., Lamont, D., & Craft, A. W. (2001). Implications of childhood obesity for adult health: Findings from thousand families cohort study. *British Medical Journal, 323*(7324), 1280–1284.

Yanovski, S. Z., & Yanovski, J. A. (2011). Obesity prevalence in the United States—up, down, or sideways? *New England Journal of Medicine, 364*(11), 987–989.

Yngve, A., Bourdeaudhuij, I. D., Wolf, A., Grjibovski, A., Brug, J., Due, P., Ehrenblad, B., Elmadfa, I., Franchini, B., Klepp, K.-I., Poortvliet, E., Rasmussen, M., Thorsdottir, I., & Rodrigo, C. P. (2007). Differences in prevalence of overweight and stunting in 11-year olds across Europe: The Pro Children Study. *European Journal of Public Health, 18*(2), 126–130.

Young, I. M. (2001). Equality of whom? Social groups and judgments of injustice. *Journal of Political Philosophy, 9*(1), 1–18.

Yu, H. J. (2011). Parental communication style's impact on children's attitudes toward obesity and food advertising. *Journal of Consumer Affairs, 45*(1), 87–107.

Zerubavel, E. (1996). Lumping and splitting: Notes on social classification. *Sociological Forum, 11*(3), 421–433.

Zitek, E. M., & Hebl, M. R. (2007). The role of social norm clarity in the influenced expression of prejudice over time. *Journal of Experimental Social Psychology, 43*(6), 867–876.

INDEX